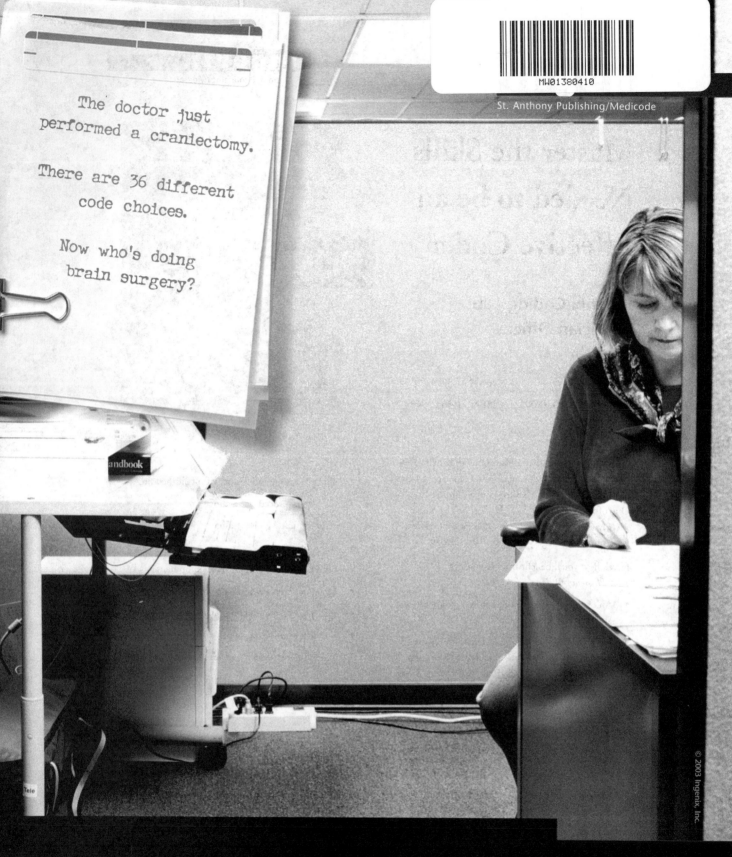

Easy-to-use solutions that simplify today's complex coding practices.

Selecting the most appropriate codes requires a working knowledge of anatomy, terminology and the nuances of different procedures. Ingenix publications and software solutions translate these procedures into clear, understandable language, with accompanying illustrations and diagrams. By taking the guesswork out of billing, compliance and reimbursement, Ingenix helps you improve operational efficiency and add to your bottom line. In short, coding never has to be a headache again. Ingenix. Simplifying the complex business of health care.

To learn more, contact us at 1-800-INGENIX, or purchase online at www.ingenixonline.com

2004 Publications

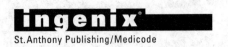

Master the Skills Needed to be an Effective Coder

Ingenix Coding Lab: Physician Offices

$74.95
Available December 2003

Item No. 5774
ISBN: 1-56337-434-X

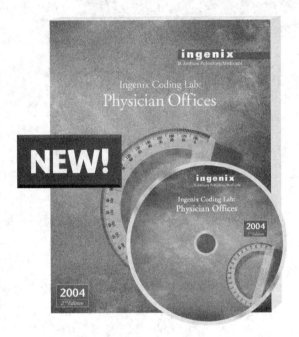

This comprehensive education module helps beginning and aspiring coders in the office or the classroom. It builds on the basics learned during Module One of *Ingenix Coding Lab: Medical Billing Basics*. *Ingenix Coding Lab: Physician Offices* was developed from our former legacy product, *Code It Right*.

Here's how you'll benefit from using *Ingenix Coding Lab: Physician Offices*:

- An excellent workbook to help you study for and pass the AAPC exam
- Help patient care staff build a solid foundation in ICD-9-CM, Physicians' Current Procedural Terminology (CPT®), and HCPCS coding
- Prepare for and pass the AAPC or AHIMA certification exams
- Make your in-house or classroom instruction more effective
- Manage coding for outpatient, long-term care, and other difficult areas
- Refine your coding and reimbursement skills to the advanced level
- Understand privacy, electronic filing, and other provisions of HIPAA

Covers:

- The profession and history of medical coding
- CPT® and procedural coding
- ICD-9 and diagnosis coding
- ICD-10
- HCPCS and durable medical equipment
- Documentation and the patient chart
- HIPAA, privacy, and compliance issues
- Public and private insurance process
- The numbers: relative values and fee schedules
- Comprehensive index, appendixes, and glossary of key terms

Also includes:

- Student workbook and free three-month subscription to *Code It Fast* on CD
- Teacher's guide on CD.

100% Money Back Guarantee:

If our merchandise* ever fails to meet your expectations, please contact our Customer Service Department toll-free at 1.800.INGENIX (464.3649), option 1, for an immediate response.

Software: Credit will be granted for unopened packages only.

CPT is a registered trademark of the American Medical Association.

SAVE 5% when you order at www.ingenixonline.com (reference source code FOBW4)

or call toll-free 1.800.INGENIX (464.3649), option 1.

Also available from your medical bookstore or distributor.

2004 Publications

Master the Skills Needed to be an Effective Coder

Ingenix Coding Lab: Facilities and Ancillary Services

$99.95 Item No. 5775
Available December 2003 ISBN: 1-56337-435-8

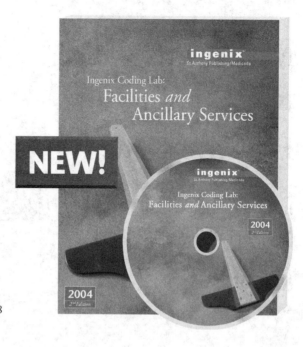

This comprehensive education module helps beginning and aspiring coders in the facility billing office or the classroom. It builds on the basics learned during Module One of *Ingenix Coding Lab: Medical Billing Basics* and Module Two of *Ingenix Coding Lab: Physician Offices*.

Here's how you'll benefit from using *Ingenix Coding Lab: Facilities and Ancillary Services*:

- Help patient care staff build a solid foundation in ICD-9-CM, Physicians' Current Procedural Terminology (CPT®), and HCPCS coding
- Prepare for and pass the AHIMA or AAPC certification exams
- Make your in-house or classroom instruction more effective
- Manage coding for outpatient, long term care, and other difficult areas
- Refine your coding and reimbursement skills to the advanced level
- Understand privacy, electronic filing, and other provisions of HIPAA

Covers:

- Hospital outpatient billing and reimbursement
- Health information management abstracting and medical documentation
- ICD-9-CM basic/intermediate diagnosis coding: Volumes I and II
- Evaluation and management coding and APCs
- Surgical CPT® coding and APCs
- Radiology CPT® coding and APCs
- Laboratory/pathology CPT® coding and APCs
- Medicine CPT® coding and APCs
- Hospital outpatient modifiers and APCs
- HCPCS Level II/DME and APCs
- Coding for ASC setting
- Comprehensive index, appendixes, and glossary of key terms
- Complex coding scenarios

Also includes:

- Student workbook and free three-month subscription to Code It Fast on CD
- Teacher's guide on CD.

100% Money Back Guarantee:

If our merchandise* ever fails to meet your expectations, please contact our Customer Service Department toll-free at 1.800.INGENIX (464.3649), option 1, for an immediate response.

*Software: Credit will be granted for unopened packages only.

CPT is a registered trademark of the American Medical Association.

SAVE 5% when you order at www.ingenixonline.com (reference source code FOBW4)

or call toll-free 1.800.INGENIX (464.3649), option 1.

Also available from your medical bookstore or distributor.

2004 Publications

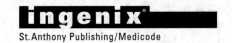

Master the Skills Needed to be an Effective Coder

Ingenix Coding Lab: Medical Billing Basics

$74.95 Item No. 5773
Available December 2003 ISBN: 1-56337-433-1

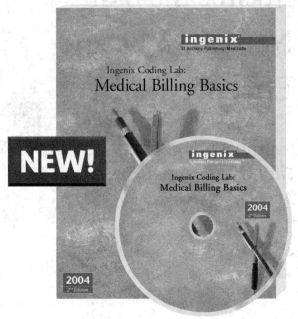

Designed to allow you to understand and master the skills needed to be an effective coder, *Ingenix Coding Lab: Medical Billing Basics*, is a comprehensive education module to help beginning and advanced coders in the office or the classroom.

Here's how you'll benefit from using *Ingenix Coding Lab: Medical Billing Basics*:

- Help patient care staff build a solid foundation in ICD-9-CM, Physicians' Current Procedural Terminology (CPT®), and HCPCS coding
- Prepare for and pass the American Academy of Professional Coders (AAPC) or American Health Information Management Association (AHIMA) certification exams
- Make your in-house or classroom instruction more effective
- Manage coding for outpatient, long term care, and other difficult areas
- Refine your coding and reimbursement skills to the advanced level
- Understand privacy, electronic filing, and other provisions of HIPAA

Covers:

- Medical terminology and human anatomy
- Insurance basics
- CPT® codes
- Diagnosis coding
- HCPCS
- Medical coding and practice management
- Inpatient coding
- ASC outpatient coding and APCs
- Coding scenarios
- Comprehensive index, appendixes, and glossary of key terms

Also includes:

- Student workbook and free three-month subscription to Code It Fast on CD
- Teacher's guide on CD

100% Money Back Guarantee:

If our merchandise* ever fails to meet your expectations, please contact our Customer Service Department toll-free at 1.800.INGENIX (464.3649), option 1, for an immediate response.

*Software: Credit will be granted for unopened packages only.

CPT is a registered trademark of the American Medical Association.

SAVE 5% when you order at www.ingenixonline.com (reference source code FOBW4)

or call toll-free **1.800.INGENIX (464.3649), option 1.**

Also available from your medical bookstore or distributor.

2004 Publications

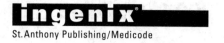
St. Anthony Publishing/Medicode

Learn to Code Easily and Accurately from Your Physician's Operative Reports

Ingenix Coding Lab: Coding from the Operative Report

$84.95 Item No. 5776
Available November 2003 ISBN 1-56337-437-4

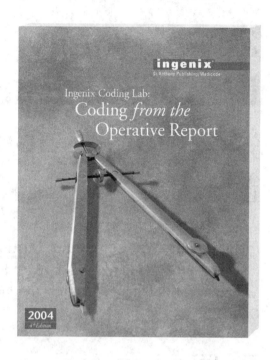

This inexpensive manual provides instruction on gleaning the proper information from physicians' documentation. Beginning with a discussion of operative reports and their importance to the coding process, the book includes examples of operative reports and operative notes, information needed to successfully and accurately code, specialty-specific scenarios, and the Physicians' Current Procedural Terminology (CPT®) chapter in which each service falls.

- **Exclusive** — The only code book dedicated to interpreting operative reports for all specialties.

- **Exclusive** — Based on real-world documentation.

- **Exclusive** — Examples based on CPT® chapters and the specialties that reside there.

- **Complete.** A comprehensive discussion of coding systems and how they're represented in operative reports.

- **Easy to Use.** Written for all levels of coder, from the beginner to the experienced professional seeking to hone skills.

- **Definitions, Key Points, Tips, and Glossaries.** Helpful tips and information throughout the book helps you select the right codes.

- **Comprehensive.** Includes most coding systems.

- **Continuing Education Units (CEUs).** Earn up to 5 CEUs through AAPC.

100% Money Back Guarantee:

If our merchandise* ever fails to meet your expectations, please contact our Customer Service Department toll-free at 1.800.INGENIX (464.3649), option 1, for an immediate response.

*Software: Credit will be granted for unopened packages only.

CPT is a registered trademark of the American Medical Association.

SAVE 5% when you order at www.ingenixonline.com (reference source code FOBW4)

or call toll-free 1.800.INGENIX (464.3649), option 1.

Also available from your medical bookstore or distributor.

FOBA 4

2004 Publications

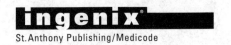

Ensure Your E/M Codes and Documentation Match!

Ingenix Coding Lab: Understanding E/M Coding (formerly Evaluation and Management Coding and Documentation Guide)

$84.95
Available: December 2003

Item No: 3186
ISBN: 1-56337-577-5

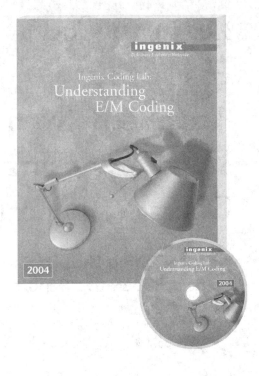

This comprehensive guide to CMS's evaluation and management (E/M) guidlines provide instructions for correctly documenting to a specific level of E/M service. Charts and templates provide excellent tools for auditing current practices and making any needed corrections. Real-world case scenarios work to help you grasp documentation requirements.

- **New—Documentation Templates.** Templates provided on diskette aid in the documentation process and help to eliminate common mistakes.

- **New—2004 Physicians' Current Procedural Terminology (CPT®) Code Changes.** Updated with the latest CPT® codes for 2004.

- **Exclusive—Self-audit Forms, Including the Official HCFA Auditing Form.** Help ensure that the documentation supports the level of E/M service coded to avoid prevent claims denials.

- **1995, 1997, and 2000 E/M Guidelines.** These guidelines prepare you for the transition to the stricter documentation requirements ahead. Allows you to see the impact these stricter guidelines will have on your practice.

- **Real-life Clinical Case Studies Updated for 2003.** Case studies iIllustrate how to apply the guidelines in everyday situations. Use them to train your staff.

- **Free—Handy E/M Fast Finder.** A portable reference organized by place of service and illustrated with tables. Practitioners can take E/M Fast Finder with them into the exam room.

- **Continuing Education Units (CEUs).** Earn 5 CEUs through AAPC.

100% Money Back Guarantee:

If our merchandise* ever fails to meet your expectations, please contact our Customer Service Department toll-free at 1.800.INGENIX (464.3649), option 1, for an immediate response.

*Software: Credit will be granted for unopened packages only.

CPT is a registered trademark of the American Medical Association.

SAVE 5% when you order at www.ingenixonline.com (reference source code FOBW4)

or call toll-free 1.800.INGENIX (464.3649), option 1.

Also available from your medical bookstore or distributor.

2004 Publications

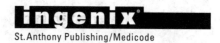
St. Anthony Publishing/Medicode

2004 ICD-9-CM Code Books for Physicians

ICD-9-CM Professional for Physicians, Vols. 1 & 2

Softbound	Compact
Item No. 5583 **$74.95**	Item No. 5587 **$69.95**
Available: September 2003	Available: September 2003
ISBN: 1-56337-474-9	ISBN: 1-56337-475-7

ICD-9-CM Expert for Physicians, Vols. 1 & 2

Spiral	Binder
Item No. 5584 **$84.95**	**$144.95**
Available: September 2003	Item No. 3534
ISBN: 1-56337-476-5	

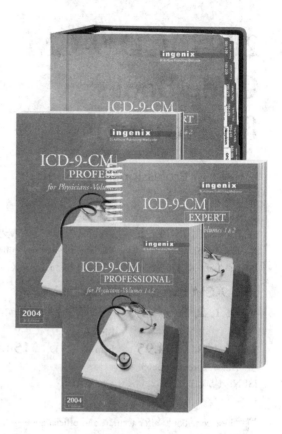

Our *ICD-9-CM for Physicians* offers easy access to pertinent coding and reimbursement information with its intuitive symbols and exclusive color coding. Plus detailed definitions and illustrations.

Professional and Expert editions feature:

- New – AHA's *Coding Clinic* for ICD-9-CM references.
- New and Revised Code Symbols.
- Fourth or Fifth-digit Alerts.
- Complete Revised Official Coding Guidelines.
- Age and Sex Edits.
- Accurate and Clear Illustrations.
- Clinically Oriented Definitions.
- Medicare as Secondary Payer Indicators.
- Manifestation Code Alert.
- Other and Unspecified Diagnosis Alerts.
- V Code Symbols. Primary and Secondary use only alerts.

The Expert editions also include these enhancements:

- **Special Reports Via E-mail.**
- **Code Tables.**
- **Valid Three-digit Category List.**

Expert Updateable Binder Subscriptions feature:

- **Three Updates a Year.** (Sept, Feb, and July)
  - Full text update with new code set in September.
  - February update with new illustrations, definitions, code edits, and AHA's *Coding Clinic* references.
  - July update newsletter with a preview of the new codes.

- **New—Summary of AHA's *Coding Clinic* Advice.** Quick look at the official advice on topics covered in the latest AHA's *Coding Clinics*.

100% Money Back Guarantee:

If our merchandise* ever fails to meet your expectations, please contact our Customer Service Department toll-free at 1.800.INGENIX (464.3649), option 1, for an immediate response.

*Software: Credit will be granted for unopened packages only.

SAVE 5% when you order at www.ingenixonline.com (reference source code FOBW4)

or call toll-free 1.800.INGENIX (464.3649), option 1.

Also available from your medical bookstore or distributor.

2004 Publications

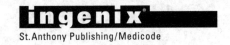
St. Anthony Publishing/Medicode

2004 ICD-9-CM Code Books for Hospitals

ICD-9-CM Professional for Hospitals, Vols. 1, 2, & 3

Softbound	Compact
Item No. 5586 **$84.95**	Item No. 5588 **$79.95**
Available: September 2003	Available: September 2003
ISBN: 1-56337-478-1	ISBN: 1-56337-479-X

ICD-9-CM Expert for Hospitals, Vols. 1, 2, & 3

Spiral	Binder
Item No. 5580 **$94.95**	Item No. 3539 **$154.95**
Available: September 2003	
ISBN: 1-56337-480-3	

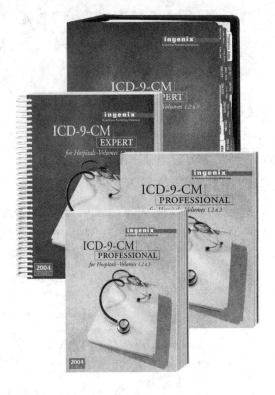

These code books offer accurate and official code information integrated with all Medicare code edits crucial to appropriate reimbursement.

Professional and Expert editions feature:

- New and Revised Code Symbols.
- Fourth or Fifth-digit Alerts.
- Complete Official Coding Guidelines
- Age and Sex Edits.
- AHA's *Coding Clinic* references.
- Illustrations and Definitions.
- Manifestation Code Alert
- Complex Diagnosis and Major Complication Alerts
- HIV Major Related Diagnosis Alert
- CC Principal Diagnosis Exclusion
- CC Diagnosis Symbol
- Crucial Medicare Procedure Code Edits

Expert editions also include these enhancements:

- **Special Reports Via E-mail**
- **PDX/MDC/DRG List**
- **Pharmacological List**
- **Valid Three-Digit Category List**
- **CC Code List**

Expert Updateable Binder Subscriptions feature:

- **Three Updates a Year.** (Sept, Feb, and July)
  - Full text update with new code set in September.
  - February update with new illustrations, definitions, code edits, and AHA's *Coding Clinic* references.
  - July update newsletter with a preview of the new codes.
- **Summary of topics covered in the the latest AHA's *Coding Clinic***

100% Money Back Guarantee:

If our merchandise* ever fails to meet your expectations, please contact our Customer Service Department toll-free at 1.800.INGENIX (464.3649), option 1, for an immediate response.

*Software: Credit will be granted for unopened packages only.

SAVE 5% when you order at www.ingenixonline.com (reference source code FOBW4)

or call toll-free 1.800.INGENIX (464.3649), option 1.

Also available from your medical bookstore or distributor.

2004 Publications

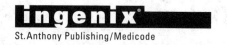
St. Anthony Publishing/Medicode

A must-have resource for ICD-9-CM users!

**ICD-9-CM Changes:
An Insider's View**

$57.95 Item No. 4952
Available: September 2003   ISBN: 1-56337-486-2

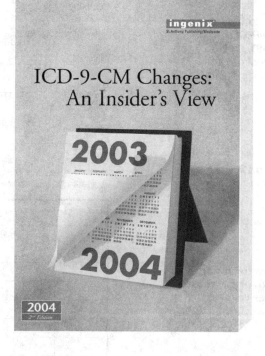

ICD-9-CM Changes: An Insider's View serves as a reference tool for understanding each of the ICD-9-CM code changes found in ICD-9-CM 2004.

Features/Benefits

- **Rationale for the New Codes and Revised Code.** Knowing the reasons behind every new or revised code change is critical to adapting coding practices.

- **Explanation of Changes to Indexes, Conventions and Instructional Notes.** Understand what other changes will impact coding practices.

- **Clinical Presentation and Treatment.** Coders must understand the clinical presentation of a condition or the intricacies of a procedure in order to code correctly without under coding or over coding.

- **Clinical Definitions of Diagnoses and Procedures.** Recognize terms found in the medical record that pertains to the new codes ensuring correct application of the code changes.

- **Coding History and Changes.** Understanding how the condition was coded in the past and how it should be coded now impacts coding practices.

- **New! Coding Scenarios.** Examples of coding scenarios clarify application the new codes.

- **Organized by Each Chapter of ICD-9-CM.** Organizing the changes in the context of relationship to other codes provides insight to the rationale of the code changes.

- **Illustrations.** Illustrations are worth a thousand words and clarify some of the complex issues surrounding many of the code changes.

- **Annotated Official Addendum.** View the official addenda that contain all the changes with annotations to the three volumes of ICD-9-CM, including text deletions.

100% Money Back Guarantee:

If our merchandise* ever fails to meet your expectations, please contact our Customer Service Department toll-free at 1.800.INGENIX (464.3649), option 1, for an immediate response.

*Software: Credit will be granted for unopened packages only.

SAVE 5% when you order at www.ingenixonline.com (reference source code FOBW4)

or call toll-free 1.800.INGENIX (464.3649), option 1.

Also available from your medical bookstore or distributor.

FOBA 4

4 Easy Ways to Order

CALL toll-free
**1.800.INGENIX
(464.3649), Option 1**
and mention the
Source Code: FOBA4

SHOP on line at
www.Ingenixonline.com

MAIL this form with
payment and/or purchase
order to:
PO Box 27116
Salt Lake City, UT 84127-0116

FAX this order form with
credit card information and /or
purchase order to 801.982.4033

Customer Service Hours
7:00am to 5:00pm MT
9:00am to 7:00pm ET

100% Money Back Guarantee

If our merchandise* ever fails to meet your expectations, please contact our Customer Service Department toll-free at 1.800.INGENIX (464.3649), Option 1 for an immediate response. We will resolve any concern without hesitation.

*Software: Credit will be granted for unopened packages only.

Shipping and Handling	
No. of Items	Fee
1	$10.95
2-4	$12.95
5-7	$14.95
8-10	$19.95
11+	Call

PUBLICATION ORDER AND FAX FORM

FOBA3

Customer No._____   Contact No._____

Purchase Order No._____   Source Code_____
(Attach copy of Purchase Order)

Contact Name _____   Title_____

Company_____

Address_____
(no P.O. Boxes, please)

City_____ State_____ Zip_____

Phone (_____)_____   Fax (_____)_____
(in case we have questions about your order)

IMPORTANT: E-MAIL REQUIRED FOR ORDER CONFIRMATION AND SELECT PRODUCT DELIVERY.
E-mail _____

Ingenix respects your right to privacy. We will not sell or rent your e-mail address or fax number to anyone outside Ingenix and its business partners. If you would like to remove your name from Ingenix promotions, please call 1.800.INGENIX (464.3649), Option 1.

Item #	Qty	Item Description	Price	Total
~~4025~~	~~1~~	~~(SAMPLE) DRG Guidebook~~	~~$89.95~~	~~$89.95~~
		Sub Total		
		TX, UT, OH, and VA residents please add applicable sales tax		
		Shipping & handling (see chart)		
		(11 plus items, foreign and Canadian orders, please call for shipping costs)		
		Total enclosed		

Payment Options
❏ Check enclosed. (Make payable to Ingenix, Inc.)
❏ Charge my: ❏ MasterCard ❏ VISA ❏ AMEX ❏ Discover
Card # | | | | | | | | | | | | | | | | Exp. Date: | | | |
                                                                                 MM   YR
❏ Bill Me P.O.#_____
Signature _____

©2003 Ingenix, Inc. All prices subject to change without notice.   FOBA4

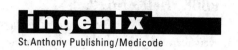

Ingenix Coding Lab:
Understanding Modifiers

2004

PUBLISHER'S NOTICE

Ingenix Coding Lab: Understanding Modifiers is designed to be an accurate and authoritative source regarding coding and every reasonable effort has been made to ensure accuracy and completeness of the content. However, Ingenix, Inc. makes no guarantee, warranty, or representation that this publication is accurate, complete, or without errors. It is understood that Ingenix, Inc. is not rendering any legal or other professional services or advice in this publication and that Ingenix, Inc. bears no liability for any results or consequences that may arise from the use of this book. Please address all correspondence to:

Ingenix Publishing Group
2525 Lake Park Blvd
West Valley City, UT 84120

AMERICAN MEDICAL ASSOCIATION NOTICE

CPT codes, descriptions, and other CPT material only are copyright ©2003 American Medical Association. All Rights Reserved. No fee schedules, basic units, relative values, or related listings are included in CPT. AMA does not directly or indirectly practice medicine or dispense medical services. AMA assumes no liability for data contained or not contained herein.

The responsibility for the content of any "Correct Coding Policy" included in this product is with the Centers for Medicare and Medicaid Services (CMS) and no endorsement by the AMA is intended or should be implied. The AMA disclaims responsibility for any consequences or liability attributable to or related to any use, nonuse, or interpretation of information contained herein.

CPT is a registered trademark of the American Medical Association.

ACKNOWLEDGMENTS

Kimberly Fisher, *Product Manager*
Elizabeth Boudrie, *Vice President, Regulatory Services*
Sheri Poe Bernard, CPC, *Director, Essential Regulatory Products*
Lynn Speirs, *Senior Director, Publishing Services Group*
Karen Schmidt, BSN, *Technical Director*

Nannette Orme, CPC, *Technical Editor*
Ms. Orme has more than 10 years of experience in the health care profession. She has extensive background in CPT/HCPCS and ICD-9-CM coding. She recently served several years as a consultant with PricewaterhouseCoopers. Her areas of expertise include physician audits and education, compliance and HIPAA legislation, litigation support for Medicare self-disclosure cases, hospital chargemaster maintenance, and emergency department coding. Ms. Orme has presented at national professional conferences and contributed articles for several professional publications. She is a member of the American Academy of Professional Coders (AAPC) and the Utah Medical Group Management Association (UMGMA).

Deborah C. Hall, CPC, *Technical Editor*
Ms. Hall is a senior clinical/technical editor for Ingenix. Ms. Hall has more than 20 years of experience in the health care field. Her experience includes 10 years as office manager for large multispecialty medical practices. Ms. Hall has written several multispecialty newsletters and coding and reimbursement manuals, and served as a health care consultant. She has taught seminars on CPT/HCPCS and ICD-9-CM coding and physician fee schedules.

Kate Holden, *Copy Editor*
Stacy Perry, *Desktop Publishing Manager*
Irene Day, *Desktop Publishing Specialist*

COPYRIGHT

©2003 Ingenix, Inc.
Printed in the United States of America.
ISBN 1-56337-436-6

Contents

Introduction 1
   What Are HCPCS Modifiers? 1
   Outpatient Modifier Guidelines/Usage 3
   Modifiers and CPT Section to Which They Apply 7

Chapter 1: Evaluation and Management 9
   21   Prolonged evaluation and management services 9
   24   Unrelated E/M service by the same physician during a postoperative period 10
   25   Significant separately identifiable E/M service by the same physician on the same day of the procedure or other service 13
   32   Mandated services 16
   52   Reduced services 18
   57   Decision for surgery 19

Chapter 2: Anesthesia 25
   23   Unusual anesthesia 25
   32   Mandated services 26
   47   Anesthesia by surgeon 26
   51   Multiple procedures 27
   53   Discontinued procedure 28
   59   Distinct procedural service 29
   Other Anesthesia Modifiers 31

Chapter 3: Surgery 33
   22   Unusual procedural services 33
   26   Professional component 35
   32   Mandated services 36
   47   Anesthesia by surgeon 37
   50   Bilateral procedure 38
   51   Multiple procedures 40
   52   Reduced services 43
   53   Discontinued procedure 44
   54   Surgical care only 46
   55   Postoperative management only 48
   56   Preoperative management only 50
   58   Staged or related procedure or service by the same physician during the postoperative period 51
   59   Distinct procedural service 53
   62   Two surgeons 55
   63   Procedure performed on infants less than 4kg 58
   66   Surgical team 59
   76   Repeat procedure by same physician 60
   77   Repeat procedure by another physician 61
   78   Return to operating room for a related procedure during the postoperative period 62
   79   Unrelated procedure or service by the same physician during the postoperative period 65

©2003 Ingenix, Inc.
CPT only ©2003 American Medical Association. All Rights Reserved.

iii

Ingenix Coding Lab: Understanding Modifiers

80 Assistant surgeon 66
81 Minimum assistant surgeon 68
82 Assistant surgeon (when a qualified resident is not available) 68
99 Multiple modifiers 70

Chapter 4: Radiology 71
22 Unusual procedural services 71
26 Professional component 72
32 Mandated services 74
50 Bilateral Procedure 74
51 Multiple procedures 75
52 Reduced services 76
53 Discontinued procedure 77
58 Staged or related procedure or service by the same physician during
   the postoperative period 79
59 Distinct procedural service 80
76 Repeat procedure by same physician 81
77 Repeat procedure by another physician 82
99 Multiple modifiers 83

Chapter 5: Pathology and Laboratory 85
22 Unusual procedural services 85
26 Professional component 86
32 Mandated services 87
52 Reduced services 87
53 Discontinued procedure 88
59 Distinct procedural service 89
90 Reference (outside) laboratory 91
91 Repeat clinical diagnostic laboratory test 91

Chapter 6: Medicine 93
22 Unusual services 93
26 Professional component 94
32 Mandated services 96
50 Bilateral procedure 96
51 Multiple procedures 97
52 Reduced services 99
53 Discontinued procedure 100
55 Postoperative management only 101
56 Preoperative management only 103
57 Decision for surgery 103
58 Staged or related procedure or service by the same physician during
   the postoperative period 104
59 Distinct procedural service 105
76 Repeat procedure by same physician 107
77 Repeat procedure by another physician 108
78 Return to operating room for a related procedure during the postoperative period 108
79 Unrelated procedure or service by the same physician during the postoperative period 110
99 Multiple modifiers 110

©2003 Ingenix, Inc.
CPT only ©2003 American Medical Association. All Rights Reserved.

iv

Contents

Chapter 7: HCPCS Modifiers A-V **113**
Introduction 113
Ambulance Modifiers 113
HCPCS Level II Modifiers 114

Chapter 8: ASC and Hospital Outpatient Modifiers **131**
Ambulatory Payment Classifications 131
Outpatient Code Editor for Outpatient Prospective Payment System 132
CPT and HCPCS Modifier Reporting Requirements 135
25   Significant separately identifiable E/M service by the same physician on
     the same day of the procedure or other service 137
27   Multiple outpatient hospital E/M encounters on the same date 138
50   Bilateral procedure 139
52   Reduced services 139
58   Staged or related procedure or service by the same physician during the
     postoperative period 140
59   Distinct procedural service 140
73   Discontinued outpatient hospital/ambulatory surgery center (ASC)
     procedure prior to the administration of anesthesia 141
74   Discontinued outpatient hospital/ambulatory surgery center (ASC)
     procedure after administration of anesthesia 141
76   Repeat procedure by same physician 142
77   Repeat procedure by another physician 142
78   Return to the operating room for a related procedure during the postoperative period 143
79   Unrelated procedure or service by the same physician during the postoperative period 143
91   Repeat clinical diagnostic laboratory test 143
HCPCS Level II Modifiers 144

Chapter 9: Modifiers and Compliance **147**
Introduction 147
What Is Compliance? 147
The OIG's Compliance Plan Guidance 150
Modifiers and Compliance: A Quick Self-Test 152

Chapter 10: Modifier Descriptors **187**

©2003 Ingenix, Inc.
CPT only ©2003 American Medical Association. All Rights Reserved.

v

Introduction

Over the last 15 to 20 years, physicians and hospitals have learned that coding and billing are inextricably entwined processes. Coding provides the common language through which the physician and hospital can communicate—or bill—their services to third-party payers, including managed care organizations, the federal Medicare program, and state Medicaid programs.

The use of modifiers is an important part of coding and billing for health care services. Modifier use has increased as various commercial payers, who in the past did not incorporate modifiers into their reimbursement protocol, recognize and accept HCPCS codes appended with these specialized billing flags.

Correct modifier use is also an important part of avoiding fraud and abuse or noncompliance issues, especially in coding and billing processes involving the federal and state governments. One of the top 10 billing errors determined by federal, state, and private payers involves the incorrect use of modifiers.

WHAT ARE HCPCS MODIFIERS?

A modifier is a two-digit numeric or alphanumeric character reported with a HCPCS code, when appropriate.

Modifiers are designed to give Medicare and commercial payers additional information needed to process a claim. This includes HCPCS Level I (Physicians' Current Procedural Terminology [CPT®]) and HCPCS Level II codes.

A modifier provides the means by which a physician or facility can indicate or "flag" a service provided to the patient that has been altered by some special circumstance(s), but for which the basic code description itself has not changed.

The CPT code book, *CPT 2004*, lists the following examples of when a modifier may be appropriate (this list does not include all of the applications for modifiers, and is provided here as part of the introductory chapter to *Ingenix Coding Lab: Understanding Modifiers*):

- A service or procedure has both a professional and technical component, but both components are not applicable
- A service or procedure was performed by more than one physician and/or in more than one location
- A service or procedure has been increased or reduced
- Only part of a service was performed
- An adjunctive service was performed
- A bilateral procedure was performed
- A service or procedure was performed more than once
- Unusual events occurred during a procedure or service
- Physical status of a patient for the administration of anesthesia

---

©2003 Ingenix, Inc.
CPT only ©2003 American Medical Association. All Rights Reserved.

CPT is a registered trademark of the American Medical Association.

Ingenix Coding Lab: Understanding Modifiers

Appendix A of *CPT 2004*, located in the back of the CPT code book, lists the 31 modifiers valid for use with the CPT codes by physicians and health care professionals, and the 13 HCPCS Level I (CPT) modifiers valid for use with CPT codes for ambulatory surgery centers (ASCs) and outpatient hospital departments. Six anesthesia physical status modifiers are also listed in the appendix. Appendix A also lists the current HCPCS Level II modifiers to be reported by ASCs and hospital outpatient departments, valid with the appropriate CPT or HCPCS Level II codes. However, it is not a complete listing of the HCPCS Level II modifiers for physicians' and other health care professionals' reporting.

The entire list of modifiers in *CPT 2004* are contained in appendix A instead of being listed in the instructional guidelines that typically precede each section of the CPT manual (e.g., evaluation and management (E/M) codes, anesthesia, surgery, etc.). To some coders this may infer an unrestricted application of the modifiers with all CPT codes. However, there are limitations for the reporting of certain modifiers with specific CPT codes. For instance, modifier 57, decision for surgery, can only be appended to appropriate E/M codes and certain ophthalmological service codes found in the medicine chapter of CPT.

Placement of a modifier after a CPT or HCPCS code does not ensure reimbursement. A special report may be necessary if the service is rarely provided, unusual, variable or new. The special report should contain pertinent information and an adequate definition or description of the nature, extent, and need for the procedure/service. The report should also describe the complexity of the patient's symptoms, pertinent history and physical findings, diagnostic and therapeutic procedures, final diagnosis and associated conditions, and follow-up care.

Some modifiers are informational only (e.g., 24 and 25) and do not affect reimbursement. They can, however, determine if the service will be reimbursed or denied.

Other modifiers such as modifier 22 (unusual procedural services) will increase the reimbursement under the protocol for many third-party payers if documentation supports the use of this modifier. Modifier 52 (reduced services) will usually equate to a reduction in payment.

There are three levels of modifiers within the HCPCS coding system. Level I (CPT) and Level II (HCPCS Level II) modifiers are applicable nationally for many third-party payers and all Medicare Part B claims. Level I or CPT modifiers are developed by the American Medical Association (AMA). HCPCS Level II modifiers are developed by the Centers for Medicare and Medicaid Services (CMS). Level III modifiers and codes were unique to each Medicare Part B carrier. The Health Insurance Portability and Accountability Act (HIPAA) guidelines indicate that all codes and modifiers are to be standardized. The Level III HCPCS codes and modifiers will be phased out as of January 2004.

There will be times when the coding and modifier information issued by CMS differs from the AMA's coding advice in the CPT manual. A clear understanding of the payers' rules is necessary in order to assign the modifier correctly.

For example, in general, a surgical service involves an evaluation of the patient by the physician prior to surgery, the surgery itself, and the postoperative follow-up care.

©2003 Ingenix, Inc.
CPT only ©2003 American Medical Association. All Rights Reserved.

Included in the CPT code book definition of a package for surgical services is the typical postoperative follow-up care." The AMA does not further define the postoperative period in the CPT code book by indicating an appropriate number of postoperative days for each procedure.

CMS and most other payers have segmented surgical procedures into major, minor, or endoscopic surgery and Medicare has its own definition of a global surgical package. To complicate matters further, the global package for a major surgery differs from that of a minor surgery. For example, the package of services for major surgery includes preoperative visits after the decision has been made to perform surgery, the intraoperative services, complications following surgery that do not require a return to the operating room, postoperative visits within 90 days after surgery, postsurgical pain management, supplies, and other miscellaneous services such as dressing changes. Medicare includes all defined services related to the surgical procedure in the amount reimbursed to the provider, including complications not requiring a return to the operating room.

The postoperative period is an amount of time following a procedure that is considered included in the reimbursement for the surgery. In other words, when a physician is paid for a particular surgery, he or she is also paid for a designated amount of time after the surgery in which he or she continues to treat the patient in follow-up visits related to the surgery. Payment for services not requiring a return to the operating room during the postoperative period is considered included in the initial reimbursement. Under Medicare guidelines the 90-day postoperative period for a major surgery includes all routine care of the patient for surgery-related services. These services should not be separately billed to Medicare for reimbursement. Medicare has three different postoperative periods for procedures performed: zero days, 10 days, and 90 days. A listing of global period assignment for procedures can be found in the *Medicare Physician Fee Schedule Database (MPFSDB).*

The appropriate use of modifier 57 can be confusing at times because Medicare's definition of this modifier differs from that of the AMA's as found in the *CPT 2003* code book. While the CPT code book simply defines it as a modifier to represent an E/M service that resulted in the initial decision to perform surgery, Medicare states that it should be used to indicate that the E/M service performed the day before or the day of surgery resulted in the decision for major surgery.

Even though CMS sets national guidelines, individual carriers are allowed to interpret many of these guidelines for their own region. This means that services/procedures allowed by one carrier may not be allowed by another. Check with your Medicare provider manual and carrier newsletters for regional determinations.

OUTPATIENT MODIFIER GUIDELINES/USAGE

CMS, through hospital transmittal number 726, dated January 1998, initially identified CPT and HCPCS Level II modifiers for hospital use when billing outpatient services (effective date July 1, 1998). Modifiers are required to ensure payment accuracy, coding consistency and editing under the outpatient prospective payment system (OPPS). The modifiers will be reported as an attachment to the HCPCS code as reported in the UB-92 form locator (FL) 44. For example, a bilateral nasal sinus endoscopy with total ethomoidectomy would be reported as 31255-50.

©2003 Ingenix, Inc.
CPT only ©2003 American Medical Association. All Rights Reserved.

Ingenix Coding Lab: Understanding Modifiers

Contents

Organization

Ingenix Coding Lab: Understanding Modifiers is a reference for physicians and their staff as well as for billers and coders of hospital outpatient services and ASC services. It includes sections that will help physicians or facility coders validate medical record documentation to support the appropriate use of the assigned modifier(s). It also includes a final section that details compliance issues as they relate to modifier reporting.

Each section lists the modifier with its precise definition. For each modifier, guidelines are provided in the following format:

- Using the modifier correctly
- Incorrect use of the modifier
- Coding tips
- Clinical examples (when appropriate)

The clinical examples provided illustrate correct modifier usage. For additional guidance, logic trees have been developed for each modifier to help determine which modifier should be applied in various situations. The logic trees can be found in "Modifiers and Compliance" in this book.

To assist in modifier application and billing, Appendix A lists the modifiers for physician and other health care professional use, as well as the "Modifiers Approved for Ambulatory Surgery Center (ASC) Hospital Outpatient Use," as described in the *CPT 2004* code book. Considering the latter modifiers, where federal information is currently available, the CMS guidelines are provided as well.

Determining Correct Use

Determining correct modifier assignment can be very frustrating at times. If the medical record documentation does not support the use of a specific modifier the physician risks denial of the claim based on lack of medical necessity and possible fraud and/or abuse penalties if/when the medical record documentation is reviewed by federal, state, and other third-party payers.

When using this book, it is important to validate the final modifier determination against the medical record documentation. First the special circumstance must be identified in the medical record. Keep in mind, a modifier provides the means by which a physician or facility can indicate that a service provided to the patient has been altered by some special circumstance(s) but the code description itself has not changed. There should be pertinent information and adequate definition of the service or procedure performed that supports the use of the assigned modifier. If the service is not documented, or the special circumstance is not indicated, it is not considered appropriate to report the modifier.

Outdated versions of CPT may include instructions for using a five-character format for reporting modifiers. To be compliant with HIPAA guidelines, the current field length of the electronic format that holds a modifier is limited to two characters.

After verifying the medical record documentation for information that supports the use of a particular modifier, then turn to the appropriate chapter of *Ingenix Coding Lab: Understanding Modifiers*. Physicians and other health care professionals will

KEY POINT

Physicians:
- Use the first seven sections of this book.

Hospital outpatient:
- Use "ASC and Hospital Outpatient Modifiers" and information found in margins throughout the book.

KEY POINT

Verify use of the modifier against the documentation.

locate the correct modifier for example, ASCs and hospital outpatient departments will find their resources in the section "ASC and Hospital Outpatient Modifiers." Pointers for correct and incorrect usage are provided for each modifier to help guide the coder and/or biller in making the right choices. For further clarification on correct modifier usage, the coder can read the clinical example(s) and check the appropriate logic tree in the "Modifiers and Compliance" section to help determine which modifier should be applied. Finally, using all available information, the coder can make a determination as to which modifier, if any, should be reported to aptly describe the service(s) rendered.

A 'How To' Example

In this example, after reviewing the patient's medical record, it is determined that the physician provided an E/M service prior to performing the surgical procedure that resulted in the decision for the surgery.

Given this documented circumstance, modifier 57 is chosen for possible assignment to the E/M code. The page for this modifier may be found in the table of contents under "Evaluation and Management." Once the modifier is located in the manual, the decision-making process can begin for correctly applying the modifier.

57   DECISION FOR SURGERY

Using the Modifier Correctly

- Add modifier 57 to the appropriate level of E/M service that resulted in the initial decision to perform the surgery.
- For Medicare claims, the 57 modifier should be used only in cases in which the decision for surgery was made during the preoperative period of a surgical procedure with a 90-day postoperative period (i.e., major surgery). The preoperative period is the day before and the day of the surgical procedure.

Incorrect Use of the Modifier

- Because of Medicare's requirements, this modifier is often misused by reporting it with an E/M service performed on the same day as a minor procedure. Do not use modifier 57 for a E/M visit furnished during the preoperative period of a minor surgical procedure (defined by Medicare as having a zero- or 10-day postoperative period). According to Medicare rules, the global surgical package for minor surgeries does not include the day prior to surgery.
- Again, under Medicare rules, this modifier is incorrectly applied by attaching it to the hospital visit code the day before surgery or the day of surgery when the decision to perform the major surgical procedure was actually made well in advance of the surgery.

Coding Tips

- A clear understanding of the payers' rules is necessary in order to assign this modifier correctly. The CPT code book simply defines 57 as a modifier to represent an E/M service that resulted in the initial decision to perform surgery. Medicare states it should be used to indicate that the E/M service performed the day before or the day of surgery resulted in the decision for major (i.e., those with a 90-day follow-up period) surgery. Medicare guidelines instruct coders to use modifier 25 if the decision for surgery is made on the same day as a minor (i.e., those with a zero- or 10-day follow-up period) or diagnostic procedure.

©2003 Ingenix, Inc.
CPT only ©2003 American Medical Association. All Rights Reserved.

- CPT codes for use with modifier 57 (unless limited by the payer) are E/M Codes 92002–92014 and 99201–99499 and ophthalmological E/M codes 92002–92004 and 92012–92014.
- This modifier is one of a group of CPT modifiers (24, 25, 57, 58, 78, and 79) that serve to identify an E/M or opthalmological service furnished during a global surgical period that is normally not a part of the global surgery package.

Clinical Example

This 75-year-old white male, well-known to the hospital GI clinic, collapsed in the waiting room. He was brought into an exam room, vomiting bloody emesis en route. An electrocardiogram was performed and interpreted as negative for acute changes, but a Q wave was noted, indicative of a previous myocardial infarction (MI). He awakened after several minutes. The patient states he has noted bloody stools for two days but today experienced moderately severe abdominal pain followed by more bloody bowel movements. He is currently responding to IV fluids.

Past Medical History: The patient has a history of gastritis, hypertension, kidney stones, urinary retention, arthritis, and elevated blood lipids. He has had bladder surgery and transurethral resection.

He is on Voltaren, Norflex, gemfibrozil for glucose intolerance and hydrochlorothiazide and had recent cortisone injections for back pain.

He is allergic to penicillin and sulfa.

Family History: Positive for diabetes mellitus (adult onset), cardiovascular heart disease and stomach CA.

Review of Systems: The patient has no urinary symptoms at this time. He does have multiple joint pains on a regular basis. The patient reports decreased vision in his left eye, possibly due to cataract. He reports shortness of breath on exertion. The patient has noted easy bruising and decreased appetite. There is no history of thyroid disease. He reports memory lapses at times but attributes this to age. The patient does not drink or smoke and is retired.

He has lost 10 pounds in the past two weeks.

He is hard of hearing in his left ear and this has been getting worse of late. He is very weak and apprehensive. He is aware of his surroundings and oriented to time and place. All other systems negative.

Physical Examination: Gray-haired, white male lying on exam table. He is diaphoretic, shaking and pale. Bp: 122/88. HEENT: within normal limits. Sclerae slightly injected. Fresh blood and vomitus debris noted in oropharynx. Some retinal changes secondary to age. No gross macular degeneration. Neck nontender. No JVD; no bruit. Thyroid: no nodule or enlargement. Heart: tachycardic at 160. No murmur or rub. Lungs: clear in all fields; shallow, rapid breathing. Abdomen: tenderness over epigastrium, referred to all quadrants with light palpation. No hepatosplenomegaly. BS: hyperactive with borborygmi. No hernia. Genitalia: normal male. Extremities: cool and clammy. Normal pulses. Neurosensory: within normal limits. Lymph: within normal limits.

Stat Labs: Pending.

Assessment:

(1) Actively bleeding peptic ulcer, moderate to severe at this time.

(2) Chronic gastritis, refractory to conservative therapies.

Plan: Fluid replacement STAT. As this is a well-known patient, the extent and severity of his peptic ulcer disease is already confirmed. Isolation of the source of hemorrhage and control of bleeding will be the primary objectives. The patient is to be admitted.

Additional information is added to the patient's medical record to reflect the postoperative diagnosis and the final procedure(s) performed, as in:

Postoperative Diagnosis: Active bleeding ulcers, multiple, 2 cm to 4 cm in diameter, adjacent to pyloric sphincter.

Procedure(s) Performed: Partial distal gastrectomy with gastroduodenostomy.

Report CPT codes 99223-57, 43631 (90-day global surgical period for Medicare patients) and 93010 (EKG interpretation). The 57 modifier is correctly appended to the hospital admission code because the decision for (major) surgery was undertaken during the admission process.

MODIFIERS AND CPT SECTION TO WHICH THEY APPLY

Modifier	Brief Description	Applicable Sections
21	Prolonged evaluation and management services	E/M
22	Unusual procedural services	Surgery, Radiology, Pathology & Laboratory, Medicine
23	Unusual anesthesia	Anesthesia
24	Unrelated E/M service by same physician during a postoperative period	E/M
25	Significant, separately identifiable E/M service by the same physician on the same day of the procedure or other service	E/M
26	Professional component	Surgery, Radiology, Pathology & Laboratory, Medicine
27*	Multiple OP hospital E/M encounters on same day	E/M
32	Mandated services	E/M, Anesthesia, Surgery, Radiology, Pathology & Laboratory, Medicine
47	Anesthesia by surgeon	Anesthesia, Surgery
50	Bilateral procedure	Surgery, Radiology, Medicine
51	Multiple procedures	Anesthesia, Surgery, Radiology, Medicine
52	Reduced services	E/M, Surgery, Radiology, Pathology & Laboratory, Medicine
53	Discontinued procedure	Anesthesia, Surgery, Radiology, Pathology & Laboratory, Medicine
54	Surgical care only	Surgery

©2003 Ingenix, Inc.
CPT only ©2003 American Medical Association. All Rights Reserved.

Ingenix Coding Lab: Understanding Modifiers

Modifier	Brief Description	Applicable Sections
55	Postoperative management only	Surgery, Medicine
56	Preoperative management only	Surgery, Medicine
57	Decision for surgery	E/M, Medicine
58	Stated or related procedure or service by the same physician during the postoperative procedure	Surgery, Radiology, Medicine
59	Distinct procedural service	Anesthesia, Surgery, Radiology, Pathology & Laboratory, Medicine
62	Two surgeons	Surgery
63	Procedure performed on infants less than 4kg	Surgery
66	Surgical team	Surgery
73*	Discontinued OP procedure prior to anesthesia administration	Anesthesia, Surgery, Radiology, Pathology & Laboratory
74*	Discontinued OP procedure after anesthesia administration	Anesthesia, Surgery, Radiology, Pathology & Laboratory
76	Repeat procedure by same physician	Surgery, Radiology, Medicine
77	Repeat procedure by another physician	Surgery, Radiology, Medicine
78	Return to the operating room for a related procedure during the postoperative period	Surgery, Medicine
79	Unrelated procedure or service by the same physician during the postoperative period	Surgery, Medicine
80	Assistant surgeon	Surgery
81	Minimum Assistant Surgeon	Surgery
82	Assistant Surgeon (when qualified resident surgeon not available)	Surgery
90	Reference (outside) laboratory	Pathology & Laboratory
91	Repeat clinical diagnostic laboratory test	Pathology & Laboratory
99	Multiple modifiers	Surgery, Radiology, Medicine

* Outpatient and ambulatory surgery center use only

Chapter 1: Evaluation and Management

21   Prolonged Evaluation and Management Services

When the face-to-face or floor/unit service(s) provided is prolonged or otherwise greater than that usually required for the highest level of evaluation and management service within a given category, it may be identified by adding modifier 21 to the evaluation and management code number. A report may also be appropriate.

Using the Modifier Correctly
- Use only with the highest level of E/M code (i.e., 99205, 99215, 99220, 99223, 99233, 99236, 99245, 99255, 99263, 99275, 99285, 99303, 99313, 99323, 99333, 99345, 99350, 99381, 99382, 99383, 99384, 99385, 99386, 99387, 99391, 99392, 99393, 99394, 99395, 99396, and 99397).
- Use modifier 21 when the face-to-face or floor/unit service provided is prolonged or otherwise greater than usually required for the highest level of E/M service within a given category. Submit a report as appropriate.
- When reporting more than 30 minutes of prolonged direct (face-to-face) patient contact, it may be more appropriate to use codes 99354–99357 in lieu of modifier 21. See the key point on this page for additional information.

Incorrect Use of the Modifier
- Placing it on all levels of E/M codes
- Placing this modifier on codes outside the code range 99205–99397 or on critical care services (99291–99292) and neonatal intensive care (99295–99296), as these services are based on units of time.

Coding Tips
- Use modifier 21 to report a service greater than that described in the highest level E/M service code. However, many third-party payers consider this modifier to be informational only (i.e., no additional payment is provided). For example, the use of 21 on the E/M code has no effect on Medicare payment.
- If the provider documented all criteria for a comprehensive service (i.e., the highest level E/M code in a given category) and continued to monitor the patient beyond 30 minutes of the time stated in the code description, see the prolonged services codes (99354–99357) in the CPT code book. Prolonged services codes are adjunctive codes for which additional reimbursement is considered and are billed with any level of E/M code.

Clinical Examples

Example #1:
A 78-year-old diabetic patient is seen in the skilled nursing facility (SNF) by her internist for stage II decubitus ulcers with cellulitis. The patient's condition requires a revision of the treatment plan. The physician performs a detailed interval history, a comprehensive physical examination and medical decision making of moderate

Key Point
Add modifier 21 to the highest level E/M code only.

Key Point
When reporting prolonged services using codes 99354–99357, remember these basic coding criteria:
- Prolonged service of less than 30 minutes is not reported—see modifier 21
- Prolonged service of less than 15 minutes beyond the first hour or beyond the final 30 minutes is not reported
- Prolonged service codes are used to designate the total duration of physician-to-patient face-to-face time beyond the typical time of the basic service
- Prolonged service is reported in addition to the basic E/M service(s) provided, at any level
- The time spent with the patient does not have to be continuous
- Prolonged service for Medicare beneficiaries can only be reported with one of the approved E/M companion codes

complexity. Following this the physician meets with members of the patient's family to discuss treatment plans and future care.

The physician spends a total of 55 minutes with the patient and family.

Since this service was greater than that usually required for CPT code 99313 (subsequent nursing facility care), submit 99313-21.

Example #2:
A 58-year-old female patient is seen for a confirmatory opinion prior to a recommended hysterectomy for uterine fibroids. The second opinion is requested by her insurance company. The gynecologist performs a comprehensive history and physical examination, as the patient has multiple chronic conditions and risk factors.

The medical decision making was of high complexity because the physician has extensive management options to consider, and must review multiple test results and related documents with the patient. The gynecologist spends extended time counseling the patient due to her extreme fear of the surgical procedure.

Submit CPT code 99275-21-32. Modifier 21 describes a prolonged E/M service and the -32 modifier indicates a third-party payer mandated second opinion.

Example #3:
A 50-year-old-male patient was admitted to the hospital by his pulmonologist with severe chronic obstructive pulmonary disease and bronchospasm. The patient was stabilized and doing well until the third day of his hospital stay when he developed acute fever, dyspnea, left lower lobe rhonchi, and laboratory evidence of hypoxemia. The pulmonologist visited the patient and performed a detailed interval history, a comprehensive examination and medical decision making of high complexity. The pulmonologist spent 55 minutes with the patient and the visit was extended due to the patient's anxiety and the family's questions. All work was performed in the patient's room and/or on the floor/unit.

Submit CPT code 99233-21.

24   UNRELATED E/M SERVICE BY THE SAME PHYSICIAN DURING A POSTOPERATIVE PERIOD

The physician may need to indicate that an evaluation and management service was performed during a postoperative period for a reason(s) unrelated to the original procedure. This circumstance may be reported by adding modifier 24 to the appropriate level of E/M service.

Using the Modifier Correctly
- CPT codes approved by CMS for use with 24 modifier are 92012–92014 and 99201–99499.
- Append modifier 24 to the E/M code for an unrelated service, for either major or minor surgical procedures.
- When a patient is admitted to a SNF for an unrelated condition in a global period, report modifier 24 with the appropriate SNF admission code.
- A physician who is responsible for postoperative care (i.e., one who has reported modifier 55) may also use modifier 24 to report any unrelated visits.

Incorrect Use of the Modifier
- Using modifier 24 with the SNF admission code when a surgeon admits a patient to a SNF and the patient's admission is related to the surgery. This service is included in the global package and will not be paid separately. Follow individual third-party payer guidelines, as some commercial health insurance plans will pay separately for these services.
- Reporting modifier 24 with the subsequent hospital care codes (99231–99233). These services performed by the surgeon during the same hospitalization as the surgery are normally related to the surgery. Separate payment for such visits are not allowed even when billed with the 24 modifier (see coding tips) unless a different diagnosis is reported with the E/M code identifying the service as unrelated to the original procedure. Follow individual third-party payer guidelines, as some commercial health insurance plans will pay separately for these services.

Coding Tips
- Use modifier 24 to indicate that an E/M service was performed during a postoperative period for a reason(s) unrelated to the original procedure. This circumstance is reported by adding the 24 modifier to the appropriate level of E/M service. Failure to use modifier 24 when appropriate may result in the denial of the E/M service by many payers.
- Use of the 24 modifier is appropriate with CPT codes 99201–99499 and 92012–92014.
- Because CPT does not define the number of days in the postoperative period, to use modifier 24 correctly, you must know the payer's definition of the postoperative period for the surgery performed. In general, the postoperative period is an amount of time following a procedure that is considered a part of the normal postoperative management of the patient. The services performed during this time period are included in the reimbursement for the surgery. In other words, when a physician is paid for a particular surgery, he or she is also paid for a designated amount of time after the surgery in which he or she continues to treat the patient in follow-up visits related to the surgery. Payment for services not requiring a return to the operating room during the postoperative period is considered included in the initial reimbursement. For example, under Medicare guidelines the postoperative period for a major surgery (i.e., 90 days) includes all routine care of the patient for surgery-related services. These services should not be separately billed to Medicare for reimbursement.
- Medicare rules state to report modifier 24 with those E/M services provided in the postoperative period of a major or minor procedure (i.e., those with a 90- or 10-day follow-up respectively) only if the E/M service is not related to the surgical procedure. A diagnosis code that clearly identifies the reason for the E/M service as unrelated to the procedure is necessary.
- Subsequent hospital care (99231–99233) and critical care services (99291–99292) by the surgeon during the same hospitalization as the surgery may be considered related to the surgery. Separate payment for such a visit is not allowed even when billed with the 24 modifier, unless one of the following exceptions apply:
  —immunotherapy management furnished by the transplant surgeon
  —critical care services unrelated to the surgery for a seriously injured or burned patient considered critically ill or injured and requiring constant physician attendance.
  —documentation attached to the claim demonstrates that the care being provided during the inpatient visits following surgery is not related to the surgery.

 CODING AXIOM

Services not included in the global surgical package include:
- Initial consultation or evaluation by the surgeon to determine the need for surgery
- Services of other physicians unless a transfer of care has been arranged
- Visits unrelated to the patient's surgical diagnosis
- Treatment for the underlying condition or an added course of treatment that is not part of normal recovery from surgery
- Diagnostic tests and procedures
- Staged or clearly distinct surgical procedures during the postoperative period
- Treatment for postoperative complications requiring a return to the operating room
- A more extensive procedure, when a less extensive procedure fails
- Supplies, such as surgical trays, splints, and casting materials when certain surgical services are performed in the physician's office
- Immunosuppressive therapy for organ transplants
- Critical care services unrelated to the surgery for a critically injured or burned patient
- Preoperative evaluations outside of the global sugical period (implemented October 2001)

 KEY POINT

When an E/M service separate from the surgical procedure is performed during the postoperative period, the diagnosis code should differ from the surgical procedure diagnosis code.

Ingenix Coding Lab: Understanding Modifiers

 KEY POINT

When determining the extent of a global surgical period for major surgeries (i.e., those procedures with a 90-day follow-up period), use the following guidelines set forth by the *Medicare Carriers Manual* (See CMS Web-based manual, pub 100-4, chapter 12). These guidelines are likewise followed by many state Medicaid programs and other major third-party payers. First, count one day immediately prior to the day of the major surgery. Then, count the day the surgical procedure is carried out, and finally count the 90 days immediately following the day of surgery. For example:

Date of surgery: April 24, 2001

Preoperative period: April 23, 2001

Last day of postoperative period: July 23, 2001.

When determining the extent of a global surgical period for minor surgeries (i.e., those procedures with zero- to 10-day follow-up periods), use the following guidelines set forth by the *Medicare Carriers Manual* (See CMS Web-based manual, pub 100-4, chapter 12). These guidelines, as well as the above-stated major surgery guidelines, are recognized by many state Medicaid programs and other major third-party payers. First, count the day the minor surgical procedure is carried out, and then count the appropriate number of days following the date of the procedure. For example:

Date of surgery (for a procedure with a 10-day postoperative period): April 24, 2001

Last day of postoperative period: May 4, 2001.

See section 4822.A.9 and 4824.A of the *Medicare Carriers Manual* (or CMS Web-based manual, pub 100-4, chapter 12, section 40.1) for further information.

- If a surgeon admits the patient to a SNF (99301–99313) for a condition unrelated to the surgical procedure, code the appropriate level of nursing home admission and append modifier 24. Documentation should be provided and the ICD-9-CM diagnosis code(s) must show an unrelated condition.
  – In order to understand this modifier it is essential that the definition of a postoperative period is known, and that the national definition of a global surgical package, as defined by the Medicare program and also used by many other third-party payers including state Medicaid programs, is also clarified. A global surgical package includes payment for the surgical procedure(s) and services related to the surgery as follows:
  —preoperative visits—after the decision for surgery is made, beginning with the day prior to surgery (major procedures) or the day of surgery (minor procedures)
  —intraoperative services—include the usual and necessary services typically carried out during the procedure
  —complications following surgery—includes additional medical and/or surgical services performed during the postoperative period not requiring a return to the operating room
  —postoperative visits and postsurgical care related to the surgery—includes, but is not limited to the following:
    – dressing changes
    – incisional care
    – removal of sutures/staples
    – removal of lines and tubes/drains
    – cast removal
    – irrigation
    – removal of urinary catheters
  —postoperative pain management—when performed by the surgeon
  —supplies
- See modifier 58 for staged procedures and 78 and 79 for return to the OR for related and/or unrelated procedures.

Clinical Examples

Example #1:
A patient at the 80th day following a transurethral resection of the prostate (TURP) is admitted to the observation service by the surgeon who performed the procedure. The patient is complaining of abdominal pain and sharp right flank pain. A work-up confirmed a kidney stone. The surgeon decides that the patient does not require surgery.

The appropriate observation code (99218–99220) is submitted with CPT modifier 24 as well as with the ICD-9-CM diagnosis code for the kidney stone to support the observation services as unrelated to the previous TURP surgery.

Example #2:

A patient presents to the surgeon's office for a postoperative visit following a cholecystectomy. She is 35 days postsurgery. During the visit the patient expresses concern about a mole on her neck that has recently changed color and increased in size. The surgeon performs a problem-focused history and an expanded problem-focused physical exam. The medical decision making is of low complexity. The surgeon will perform a biopsy in three days.

Submit CPT code 99213-24 to describe the encounter. The diagnosis code should describe the mole and, therefore, demonstrate a different diagnosis than the one that required the cholecystectomy. (Remember for established patient office visits, only two of the three key elements must be documented in the patient's medical record.)

Example #3:

An 88-year-old patient has recovered well after her recent surgery for gallstones. Her temperature is normal, her wounds are healing well, she is able to eat soft foods and she is urinating well and having normal bowel movements. Her disposition is mercurial, however, during her hospital stay she demonstrates an inability to remember several of her family member's names, and is not oriented to time and place. These are not abrupt changes, and correlate to the surgeon's office notes. Representatives of the patient's family confirm her increasing organic brain syndrome. After discussing all options with the family and the case social worker, it is decided the patient should be admitted to a SNF upon discharge. The surgeon subsequently admits the patient to the SNF with diagnoses for organic brain syndrome with significant memory loss and moderate dementia. For this admission, the surgeon performs a comprehensive history and physical assessment and decision making of moderate complexity. A medical plan of care is created to be carried out during the patient's stay in the SNF.

Submit CPT code 99303-24.

25 SIGNIFICANT SEPARATELY IDENTIFIABLE E/M SERVICE BY THE SAME PHYSICIAN ON THE SAME DAY OF THE PROCEDURE OR OTHER SERVICE

The physician may need to indicate that on the day a procedure or service identified by a CPT code was performed, the patient's condition required a significant, separately identifiable E/M service above and beyond the other service provided or beyond the usual preoperative and postoperative care associated with the procedure that was performed. The E/M service may be prompted by the symptom or condition for which the procedure and/or service was provided. As such, different diagnoses are not required for reporting of the E/M services on the same date. This circumstance may be reported by adding the modifier 25 to the appropriate level of E/M service.

Note: This modifier is not used to report an E/M service that resulted in a decision to perform surgery. See modifier 57.

©2003 Ingenix, Inc.
CPT only ©2003 American Medical Association. All Rights Reserved.

Ingenix Coding Lab: Understanding Modifiers

KEY POINT

Medicare carriers have been instructed by CMS to conduct claim reviews to detect high use of modifier 25 by individual providers or groups. When an individual or group has been identified, a case-by-case review of all claims and supporting documentation will be performed on subsequent submissions containing modifier 25. CMS has instructed the carriers to educate the offending individual providers or groups in the appropriate use of this modifier.

QUICK TIP

Hospital ASC and Outpatient Coders

Effective October 1, 2001, Medicare clarifies that modifier 25 should be used according to the CPT definition of "significant, separately identifiable E/M service" for emergency department E/M codes. The OCE will only edit for modifier 25 when it is reported with a procedure that has a status indicator of S or T.

Status indicators under OPPS determine the payment method. Significant procedures have a status of S or T and the difference is that procedures with a T status will receive a multiple procedure discount when performed with another procedure of T status, and those with a status S will not receive a multiple procedure discount.

Under Medicare OPPS, any claim submitted with an E/M service on the same date as a procedure with an S or T status without modifier 25 will cause a line-item rejection.

Using the Modifier Correctly

- Use modifier 25 when the E/M service is separate from that required for the procedure and a clearly documented, distinct and significantly identifiable service was rendered. However, although CPT does not limit this modifier to use only with a specific type of procedure or service, many third-party payers will not accept modifier 25 on an E/M service when billed with a minor procedure on the same day.
- When using 25 on an E/M service on the same day as a procedure, the E/M service must have the key elements (history, examination, and medical decision making) well-documented.
- Use modifier 25 on initial hospital visit (CPT codes 99221–99223), an initial inpatient consultation (CPT codes 99251–99255) and a hospital discharge service (CPT codes 99238 and 99239), when billed for the same date as an inpatient dialysis service.
- Use modifier 25 when preoperative critical care codes are billed within a global surgical period. Reporting these E/M services with modifier 25 indicates that they are significant and separately identifiable services.
- Use modifier 25 on an E/M service when performed at the same session as a preventive care visit when a significant, separately identifiable E/M service is performed in addition to the preventive care. The E/M service must be carried out for a nonpreventive clinical reason, and the ICD-9-CM code(s) for the E/M service should clearly indicate the nonpreventive nature of the E/M service.
- Attach modifier 25 to the E/M code representing a significant, separately identifiable service performed on the same day as routine foot care. The visit must be medically necessary.

Incorrect Use of the Modifier

- Using modifier 25 to report an E/M service that resulted in the decision to perform major surgery (see modifier 57).
- Billing an E/M service with modifier 25 when a physician performs ventilation management in addition to an E/M service.
- Using modifier 25 on an E/M service performed on a different day than the procedure. For example, a surgeon sees a patient in his office to follow-up an abnormal mammogram. After discussing the findings with the patient, he schedules and performs a breast biopsy the next day. It would be incorrect to add modifier 25 to the E/M code.
- Using modifier 25 on a surgical code (10021–69990) since this modifier is used to explain the special circumstance of providing the E/M service on the same day as a procedure
- Using modifier 25 on the office visit E/M level of service code when on the same day a minor procedure (e.g., an endometrial biopsy) was performed, when the patient's trip to the office was strictly for the minor procedure (e.g., biopsy).

Coding Tips

- Use modifier 25 to indicate that on the day of a procedure or other service identified by a CPT code, the patient's condition required a significant, separately identifiable E/M service above and beyond the other service provided or beyond the usual preoperative and postoperative care associated with the procedure that was performed.

©2003 Ingenix, Inc.
CPT only ©2003 American Medical Association. All Rights Reserved.

Chapter 1: Evaluation and Management

- Medicare will allow separate payment for two office visits provided on the same date, by the same physician, when each visit is rendered for an unrelated problem. Both visits must occur at different times of the day and both visits must be medically necessary. This particular circumstance is considered rare, and requires modifier 25 to be appended to the second visit.

- Although the CPT code book does not limit this modifier to use only with a specific type of procedure or service, the general rule most insurance carriers follow is that they will not pay for an E/M visit and a minor procedure on the same day. Keep in mind, third-party payers may follow the CPT code book, Medicare's or their own definition of a minor procedure.

- There is a difference between the CPT code book definition and the instructions from Medicare. Medicare guidelines instruct coders to use modifier 25 if the decision for surgery is made on the same day as a minor surgery (i.e., in those with a zero- to 10-day follow-up period) or diagnostic procedure. The 57 modifier would be added to the appropriate level of E/M code when the initial decision to perform major surgery (i.e., those with a 90-day follow-up period) is made during an E/M service the day before or the day of surgery.

- Use codes 99291–99292 and modifier 25 to indicate critical care services provided during a global surgical period for a seriously injured or burned patient. These services are not considered related to a surgical procedure and are paid separately as long as the patient is critically ill and requires the constant attention of the physician, and the critical care is unrelated to the specific anatomic injury or general surgical procedure performed. Documentation that the critical care was unrelated to the specific anatomic injury or general surgical procedure performed must be submitted. Submission of an ICD-9-CM code in the range 800.0–959.9 (except 930–939) is considered acceptable documentation by most carriers.

- Medicare's relative work values for CPT codes 98925–98929, osteopathic manipulative treatment (OMT) services, include cursory history and palpatory examination. Attach CPT modifier 25 to the E/M service only if the E/M service is a significant, separately identifiable E/M service by the same physician on the day of OMT. OMT is considered to be a procedure, and an E/M service is not paid on the same day as OMT. Physicians should not upcode the E/M service and omit the code for the OMT service or report different diagnoses for the two services if both services are provided for the same reason.

- CPT codes for use with modifier 25 are 92002–92014 and 99201–99499 unless limited by the payer.

Clinical Examples

Example #1:

A patient is seen for re-evaluation of chronic refractory hypertension. The physician performs a detailed history and physical examination and medical decision making of moderate complexity. During this encounter, the patient states that he is having trouble hearing. The physician examines the patient's ears and discovers that the right ear is blocked with cerumen. After irrigation and removal of a wax plug, the patient is able to hear better. The patient's hypertension will be treated with a new medication and a re-evaluation is scheduled for one month.

In order to ensure payment of all services, the ICD-9-CM codes must be linked to the CPT codes properly. The hypertension code (401.9) would be linked to the E/M visit code and the ear irrigation procedure would be linked to the code for impacted cerumen (380.4). Submit CPT codes 99214-25 and 69210.

©2003 Ingenix, Inc.
CPT only ©2003 American Medical Association. All Rights Reserved.

15

Ingenix Coding Lab: Understanding Modifiers

Example #2:

A 33-year-old male, new patient, presents to the physician's walk-in service after sustaining a head injury while renovating his house. According to the patient, a lighting fixture fell and hit his head as he was attempting to hang it. He immediately applied compresses to the temporoparietal wound area, and had his wife drive him to the office. He reports heavy bleeding, but only shows light hemorrhage at this time. He cannot confirm loss of consciousness, but denies dizziness or blurred vision. Denies nausea or vomiting. Denies dystaxia. Does not complain of headache except in the immediate area of the wound. The patient has never had a tetanus shot.

A complete review of systems is performed, and the past medical, family and social histories are taken. The remainder of the detailed history is completed. The temporoparietal scalp wound is debrided of dried blood and blood clots. After irrigation, the cranial muscle fascia is noted through the wound. A layered closure is performed on this 5.5 cm wound. A detailed neurological evaluation is then performed to rule out increased intracranial pressure. There are no neurological signs or deficits noted. Medical decision making is of low complexity. Finally, a tetanus toxoid inoculation is administered. The signs for intracranial pressure changes are reviewed with the patient and he is given follow up instructions.

Report CPT code 99203-25 for the history, physical and medical decision making portions of the E/M visit, and report code 12032 for the layered closure of the open scalp wound. Report code 90703 for the tetanus inoculation. All services should be linked to the same ICD-9-CM code for open wound (873.0).

Example #3:

An established patient presents with uterine bleeding requiring a hysteroscopy with endometrial biopsy; the patient is also evaluated for a breast cyst. The breast evaluation consists of an expanded problem-focused history and physical exam and medical decision making of low complexity.

In this case, only the E/M elements of the visit related to the breast cyst would be used to justify the correct level of service for the office visit.

Submit CPT codes 99213-25 and 58558. The diagnosis for the breast cyst would be linked to the E/M service code (99213-25), and the diagnosis for the uterine bleeding would be linked to the hysteroscopy procedure (58558).

32   MANDATED SERVICES

Services related to mandated consultation and/or related services (e.g., QIO, third-party payer, governmental, legislative, or regulatory requirement) may be identified by adding the modifier 32 to the basic procedure.

Using the Modifier Correctly

- Use modifier 32, when the physician is aware of third-party involvement regarding mandated services.
- Modifier 32 is considered informational and, when used, many insurers allow 100 percent reimbursement without a deductible or copayment. However, modifier 32 has no effect on Medicare payment.

Chapter 1: Evaluation and Management

Incorrect Use of the Modifier

- Lack of understanding as to the intent of this modifier may lead to inappropriate assignment. Do not use this modifier when a patient or family member requests a second opinion from another physician.

Coding Tips

- Use modifier 32 to indicate mandated consultations and/or related E/M services.

- A common situation where this modifier is used would be in a workers' compensation case. Oftentimes, the insurance company paying for the services will ask the patient to see a different doctor for another opinion. The physician providing the opinion would append the 32 modifier on the consultation code (99271–99275) to indicate that a third-party requested this service.

- CPT codes for use with modifier 32 are 99201–99499, 00100–01999, 10021–69990, 70010–79999, 80048–89399, and 90281–99600 unless limited by the payer.

Clinical Examples

Example #1:

A three-year-old child is ordered by the department of family services (via the court system) to be taken to a physician that works as part of a child protection team for suspicion of child abuse. The child protection team is aware that this examination may be very frightening to the child. Great care is extended to spend time with the patient and explain as much as possible to her before the examination takes place. After an hour of letting the child play and get acquainted, it becomes apparent that she is not going to allow the examination. It is decided that conscious sedation will be appropriate in this case. The child is sedated and examined. A comprehensive history, physical and medical decision making of high complexity are performed. Photographs and lab tests are taken. The patient encounter/face-to-face physician time is 95 minutes in duration.

The E/M service performed qualifies for a level 99205, office or other outpatient visit, based on the three key elements documented in the medical record. This is reported with CPT code 99354, prolonged services, since the time requirements of 99205 have been exceeded and the criteria for reporting 99354 have been met. CPT code 99205 is appended with the 32 modifier because the E/M encounter was a mandated service. Report code 99141 or 99142 dependent upon the type of conscious sedation provided by the physician and staff.

Example #2:

A workers' compensation carrier has requested a confirmatory consultation of a 42-year-old woman, injured on the job three years ago. She worked as a machine operator in a dye casting company. The patient sustained extensive lacerations and crushing injury to the right hand after accidentally getting her hand caught in rotating machinery parts. Recent examinations have not confirmed total loss of hand function, contradicting the patient's subjective complaints. Therefore, the carrier wishes to have the patient independently evaluated prior to reducing her compensation benefits. The patient is scheduled for evaluation by an orthopaedic surgeon subspecializing in hand surgery for confirmatory opinion.

©2003 Ingenix, Inc.
CPT only ©2003 American Medical Association. All Rights Reserved.

The orthopaedic surgeon performs a comprehensive history and physical examination, and reviews all accompanying medical records and diagnostic studies. Medical decision-making is of high complexity. A written report of the findings and medical opinion are forwarded to the workers' compensation carrier.

Report CPT code 99275, appended by modifier 32 for mandated services.

52 REDUCED SERVICES

Under certain circumstances a service or procedure is partially reduced or eliminated at the physician's discretion. Under these circumstances the service provided can be identified by its usual procedure number and the addition of the modifier 52, signifying that the service is reduced. This provides a means of reporting reduced services without disturbing the identification of the basic service. **Note:** For hospital outpatient reporting of a previously scheduled procedure/service that is partially reduced or cancelled as a result of extenuating circumstances or those that threaten the well-being of the patient prior to or after administration of anesthesia, see modifiers 73 and 74.

Using the Modifier Correctly
- Use modifier 52 for reporting services that were partially reduced or eliminated at the physician's election. Documentation explaining the reduction should be present in the medical record.
- Use modifier 52 to indicate that a procedure is being performed at a lesser level. A concise statement that describes how the service differs from the normal procedure must be included on the claim or in the appropriate field for electronic claims.

Incorrect Use of the Modifier
- Using modifier 52 for terminated procedures. It is intended for procedures that accomplished some result, but less than expected for the procedure.
- Many insurance companies do not recognize the 52 modifier appended to an E/M service. In addition, time-based codes (i.e., critical care, psychotherapy, anesthesia) and automated-organ or disease-oriented panels also may have limitations on modifier usage. Check with your carriers to see if they recognize this modifier and request their policy on its use.

Coding Tips
- Use modifier 52 to indicate that under certain circumstances, a service or procedure is partially reduced or eliminated at the physician's discretion.
- The 52 modifier is for a reduced service and is not a modifier to be used when the fee is reduced as a result of a patient's inability to pay.
- This modifier, while rarely used with an E/M code, is used to report that a service was not completed in its entirety. For example, a preventive medicine visit normally requires a comprehensive history and physical examination geared to the age of the patient. This may not always be performed to the extent described by the code description. In this case, append modifier 52 to the preventive medicine code.
- CPT codes for use with modifier 52 unless limited by the payer are 99201–99499 (except for Medicare), 10021–69990, 70010–79999, 80048–89399, 90281–99600 (except psychotherapy), when appropriate.

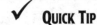

QUICK TIP

If a surgical procedure or service is terminated due to extenuating circumstances that threaten the patient's well-being, see modifier 54.

QUICK TIP

The *Medicare Carriers Manual* (See CMS Web-based manual, pub 100) states, in part, that when surgical procedures for which services performed are significantly less than usually required, [these services] may be billed with modifier 52. Surgical procedures reported with this modifier should include the following documentation:

- A concise statement about how the service or procedure differs from the usual
- The operative report

Claims reported with modifier 52 that do not include the required documentation will be processed as if there were no modifiers reported. For more information about 52 modifier reporting with surgical services, see the surgery chapter.

Chapter 1: Evaluation and Management

Clinical Examples

Example #1:
A 14-year-old boy, in apparent good health, who is an established patient in our practice, presents for a scout physical. His troop will be leaving the end of this month for a one-week stay in the mountains. He is well-groomed and polite. Reviewed safety issues with him and spoke to him about school and social issues, such as not getting involved with drugs or alcohol. I asked him if he was sexually active. He denied all of the above. No fatigue; he is active in soccer and baseball. No allergies, TD up to date. A detailed examination was then performed. His scouting papers were completed with the required information, clearing him for this club activity.

Submit CPT code 99394-52. The preventive care CPT code requires a comprehensive history and physical, and the physician elected to not perform them to the comprehensive level, as this was not medically necessary. A 52 modifier is attached to the preventive care service, alerting the insurance company that the service was reduced.

Example #2:
A patient is admitted to a SNF for senile dementia and bladder and fecal incontinence, as well as decubitus foot ulcers due to diabetes. The physician starts the initial assessment, takes a comprehensive history, but before he can complete the treatment plan and physical examination, the patient becomes adamant about leaving the facility and leaves with her family against medical advice.

Submit CPT code 99303-52.

57   DECISION FOR SURGERY

An evaluation and management service that resulted in the initial decision to perform the surgery may be identified by adding the modifier 57 to the appropriate level of E/M service.

Using the Modifier Correctly
- Add modifier 57 to the appropriate level of E/M service that resulted in the initial decision to perform the major surgery; some commercial third-party payers will accept the 57 modifier appended to E/M services that result in a decision for minor surgery.
- For Medicare claims, the 57 modifier should be used only in cases in which the decision for surgery was made during the preoperative period of a surgical procedure with a 90-day postoperative period (i.e., major surgery). The preoperative period is defined as the day before and the day of the surgical procedure.

Incorrect Use of the Modifier
- Because of Medicare's requirements, this modifier is often misused by being placed on an E/M service performed on the same day as a minor procedure. Do not use modifier 57 on the E/M visit furnished during the preoperative period of a minor procedure (defined by Medicare as having a zero- to 10-day postoperative period). According to Medicare rules, where the decision to perform the minor procedure is typically done immediately before the service, it is considered a routine preoperative service and a visit or consultation is not billed in addition to the procedure.

 QUICK TIP

The following consultation codes can be considered for reimbursement, even though they are now included in the Correct Coding Initiative (CCI) edits. These services can be eligible for payment when modifier 57 is appended to the E/M code representing the type and level of consultation rendered for the decision for surgery:

99241	99251	99271
99242	99252	99272
99243	99253	99273
99244	99254	99274
99245	99255	99275

©2003 Ingenix, Inc.
CPT only ©2003 American Medical Association. All Rights Reserved.

Ingenix Coding Lab: Understanding Modifiers

- Attaching modifier 57 to the hospital visit code for the day before surgery or day of surgery when the decision to perform the "major" surgical procedure (as defined by Medicare) was made well in advance of the surgery.

Coding Tips

- A clear understanding of the payers' rules is necessary in order to assign this modifier correctly. The CPT code book defines 57 as a modifier to represent an E/M service that resulted in the initial decision to perform surgery; Medicare states it should be used to indicate that the E/M service performed the day before or the day of surgery resulted in the decision for major surgery (i.e., those with a 90-day follow-up period). Medicare guidelines instruct coders to use modifier 25 if the decision for surgery is made on the same day as a minor surgery (i.e., in those with a zero- to 10-day follow-up period) or diagnostic procedure.
- It may be possible to use the 57 on a minor procedure. Check with your third-party payers on their definition of a "minor" procedure and whether modifier 57 can be used on such codes.
- The 57 modifier can only be appended to an E/M code and ophthalmological codes 92012 and 92014, unless limited by the payer.
- This modifier is one of a group of CPT modifiers (24, 25, 57, 58, 78 and 79) that serve to identify an E/M or certain ophthalmological service furnished during a global surgical period that is normally not a part of the global surgery package.

Clinical Examples

Example #1:

This 75-year-old white male, well-known to the hospital GI clinic, collapsed in the waiting room. He was brought into an exam room, vomiting bloody emesis en route. An electrocardiogram was performed and interpreted as negative for acute changes, but a Q wave was noted, indicative of a previous myocardial infarction (MI). He awakened after several minutes. The patient states he has noted bloody stools for two days but today experienced moderately severe abdominal pain followed by more bloody bowel movements. He is currently responding to IV fluids.

Past Medical History: The patient has a history of gastritis, hypertension, kidney stones, urinary retention, arthritis and elevated blood lipids. He has had bladder surgery and transurethral resection.

He is on Voltaren, Norflex, gemfibrozil for glucose intolerance and hydrochlorothiazide and had recent cortisone injections for back pain.

He is allergic to penicillin and sulfa.

Family History: Positive for diabetes mellitus (adult onset), cardiovascular heart disease and stomach CA.

Review of Systems: The patient has no urinary symptoms at this time. He does have multiple joint pains on a regular basis. The patient reports decreased vision in his left eye, possibly due to cataract. He reports shortness of breath on exertion. The patient has noted easy bruising and decreased appetite. There is no history of thyroid disease. He reports memory lapses at times but attributes this to age. The patient does not drink or smoke and is retired.

✓ **QUICK TIP**

A perennial favorite of Medicare and other third-party payer fraud and abuse investigation units has been the investigating of inappropriate consultation reporting. In many instances following these investigations, services inappropriately billed as consultations have been downgraded to office or other outpatient services, or hospital inpatient services. It is extremely important to recognize and document the following three basic criteria for an E/M service to qualify as a consultation:

- A request for the consultation from another physician or other appropriate source, together with the reason for the consultation, documented in the medical record
- The consultation must be requested and rendered only for the medical opinion and/or advice of the consultant, although the consultant can initiate diagnostic and/or therapeutic services during the same or subsequent visit
- The results of the consultation must be communicated back to the requesting physician or source; this communication must be in writing

The CPT manual states: "The consultant's opinion and any services that were ordered or performed must also be documented in the patient's medical record and communicated by written report to the requesting physician or other appropriate source."

©2003 Ingenix, Inc.

CPT only ©2003 American Medical Association. All Rights Reserved.

He has lost 10 pounds in the past two weeks.

He is hard of hearing in his left ear and this has been getting worse of late. He is very weak and apprehensive. He is aware of his surroundings and oriented to time and place. All other systems negative.

Physical Examination: Gray-haired, white male lying on exam table. He is diaphoretic, shaking and pale. BP 122/87. HEENT: within normal limits. Sclerae slightly injected. Fresh blood and vomitus debris noted in oropharynx. Some retinal changes secondary to age. No gross macular degeneration. Neck nontender. No JVD; no bruit. Thyroid: no nodule or enlargement. Heart: tachycardic at 160. No murmur or rub. Lungs: clear in all fields; shallow, rapid breathing. Abdomen: tenderness over epigastrium, referred to all quadrants with light palpation. No hepatosplenomegaly. BS: hyperactive with borborygmi. No hernia. Genitalia: normal male. Extremities: cool and clammy. Normal pulses. Neurosensory: within normal limits. Lymph: within normal limits.

Stat Labs: Pending.

Assessment:

(1) Actively bleeding peptic ulcer, moderate to severe at this time.

(2) Chronic gastritis, refractory to conservative therapies.

Plan: Fluid replacement STAT. As this is a well-known patient, the extent and severity of his peptic ulcer disease is already confirmed. Isolation of the source of hemorrhage and control of bleeding will be the primary objectives. The patient is to be admitted.

Following the procedure, additional information is added to the patient's medical record to reflect the postoperative diagnosis and the final procedure(s) performed, as in:

Postoperative Diagnosis: Active bleeding ulcers, multiple, 2 cm to 4 cm in diameter, adjacent to pyloric sphincter.

Procedure(s) Performed: Partial distal gastrectomy with gastroduodenostomy.

Report CPT codes 99223-57, 43631 (90-day global surgical period for Medicare patients) and 93010 (EKG interpretation). The 57 modifier is correctly appended to the hospital admission code because the decision for (major) surgery was undertaken during the admission process.

Example #2:
A Medicare patient at the 73rd day following a TURP is admitted to the observation service with abdominal pain by the surgeon who performed the procedure. The physician performs a comprehensive history and physical examination and the medical decision making is of high complexity, given the patient's age, multiple medical problems and surgical history. During this encounter, the surgeon decides that the patient will require an exploratory laparotomy. It appears this event is not related to the TURP.

Submit CPT codes 99220-24-57. The surgeon uses modifier 57 on the observation code to indicate that the decision for surgery was made on the observation day admission (the previous day). The -24 modifier is also added to indicate that the E/M service was not related to the original procedure. [**Note:** The subsequent surgical procedure, CPT code 49000, performed the next day would be reported with modifier 79 with the appropriate date of service. (See chapter 3 for more details.)]

Example #3:
A male patient is seen by a cardiologist for evaluation of chest pain. Following a positive cardiac catheterization, the cardiologist refers him to a cardiothoracic surgeon to evaluate for possible surgery. The cardiothoracic surgeon notes that the patient is 68 years old and exhibits multivessel coronary artery disease. Pulmonary artery hypertension is also identified. A pulmonologist has been treating him for this problem. His cardiac echo demonstrates pulmonary pressures in the 30 range, which had previously been in the 70 to 80 range. The surgeon performs a comprehensive history and physical examination, and admits the patient with plans to perform immediate major surgery on the following day. The surgery will consist of combined arterial-venous grafting for coronary bypass. This will involve using three venous grafts and three arterial grafts.

Submit CPT code 99223-57, 33535, and 33519. The 57 modifier is added to the E/M hospital admission code because the decision to provide surgery was made during the patient encounter and the surgery was to be performed within the preoperative period.

Example #4:
A 92-year-old female presents to the ED after falling at home and injuring her left arm and leg. She complains of wrist and knee pain. The patient is pleasant, cooperative and oriented x3. Due to the age of the patient and nature of her complaints, a complete history is taken and a detailed physical examination is performed. Examination revealed a contusion, abrasion and superficial laceration of the dorsum of the left wrist with deformity, and swelling and tenderness of the left knee without any instability or crepitus. She is on multiple medications including Lasix, Procardia, Zestril, Nitro-Dur, digoxin, and Maxzide. She has daily nursing care and a family who assists in her care.

Quick Tip

Hospital ASC and Outpatient Coders
Facilities should use 25 in place of modifier 57 for the ED visit on the same day as a procedure that has a status of indicator of S or T. Modifier 57 is not a valid hospital/ASC modifier.

The x-rays reveal no knee fracture, but she does have a nondisplaced fracture of the distal radius (Smith-type), of the left wrist. A knee immobilizer is placed. The decision is made to perform closed treatment of the distal radius fracture without manipulation. The medical decision making for this encounter is of moderate complexity. She is to follow up with her family physician early in the following week. Her diagnoses are a fracture of the left wrist with accompanying contusions and a superficial laceration, and a contusion and strain of her left knee.

Submit CPT codes: 99284-57 and 25600-54.

Note: If the ED physician interpreted the x-rays and documented this service by a written report the findings and recommendations, the physician could also bill the radiology codes with modifier 26. Only one physician can bill for an x-ray or EKG interpretation done in the ED.

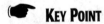

Key Point

ED physicians should append modifier 54, surgical care, only to fracture care codes when they do not provide all of the follow-up care associated with the fracture.

Example #5
The patient presents to her internist's office with complaints of abdominal pain that started the previous day. The patient complains of nausea and dry heaves. The patient

denies diarrhea, SOB or fever. The patient is sent to a general surgeon the same day for evaluation. The surgeon takes a comprehensive history and physical and notes, upon obtaining her vital signs, that she does have a slightly elevated temperature. This 89-year-old woman is status post gallbladder surgery several years ago. Her abdomen exam indicates diffuse pain with hypoactive bowel sounds. Abdomen is tender primarily in the epigastrium. The general surgeon admits the patient to the hospital for an exploratory laparotomy scheduled for the next day.

Submit CPT code 99223-57 and the surgical procedure(s) performed.

Chapter 2: Anesthesia

23   Unusual Anesthesia

Occasionally, a procedure, which usually requires either no anesthesia or local anesthesia, because of unusual circumstances must be done under general anesthesia. This circumstance may be reported by adding the modifier 23 to the anesthesia code for the basic service.

Using the Modifier Correctly
- Modifier 23 should be used on basic service procedure codes (00100–01999).
- Use this modifier when general anesthesia is administered in situations that typically would not require this level of anesthesia, or in situations in which local anesthesia might have been required, but would not be sufficient under the circumstances.
- When using modifier 23, the claim must be accompanied by both documentation and a cover letter from the physician explaining the need for general anesthesia.

Incorrect Use of the Modifier
- Appending modifier 23 to anesthesia or surgical CPT codes when billing Medicare.
- Using modifier 23 for local anesthesia.

Coding Tips
- Add modifier 23 to the procedure code for the basic service when a procedure which usually requires either no anesthesia or local anesthesia, must be done under general anesthesia because of unusual circumstances.
- CPT codes for use with modifier 23 unless limited by the payer are: 00100–01999.

Clinical Examples

Example #1

A mentally retarded, extremely anxious female patient presents to the outpatient hospital clinic for excision of a 2 cm. cystic lesion on her arm. When the physician tries to examine her, she becomes so agitated that he is unable to perform the examination. After an attempt at conscious sedation fails to calm the patient, the physician decides that an anesthesiologist must be summoned to induce general anesthesia. Since the patient has been NPO for greater than six hours, the on-call anesthesiologist is able to administer the anesthetic and the procedure is completed.

The CPT code is submitted with modifier 23 as well as HCPCS Level II modifier AA.

Example #2

An eight-year-old hyperactive child is seen in the ED with complaint of a foreign body in his left ear. It appears he pushed a round metal ball into his ear. The child is frightened and is unmanageable. The anesthesiologist is called to administer a general anesthetic so the obstructing foreign body can be extricated from the patient's ear

Key Point

Claims submitted to Medicare, Medicaid, and other third-party payers containing modifier 23 for unusual anesthesia that do not have attached supporting documentation that demonstrates the unusual distinction of the services will generally be processed as if the procedure codes were not appended with the modifier. Some third-party payers might suspend the claims and request additional information from the respective anesthesiologists, but this is the exception rather that the rule.

Quick Tip

The federal Medicare program bases its definition of concurrent medically directed anesthesia procedures on the maximum number of cases that an anesthesiologist is medically directing at one time, and whether or not these other procedures overlap one another. Concurrency is not dependent on each of the cases involving a Medicare patient, however. If an anesthesiologist directs three concurrent procedures, two of which involve non-Medicare patients and one that does involve a Medicare patient, this represents three concurrent medically directed cases. Base unit reductions for concurrent medically directed procedures will apply.

canal without damaging the patient's tympanic membrane due to the child's agitation.

The anesthesia CPT code is submitted with modifier 23 as this is an unusual circumstance.

32   MANDATED SERVICES

Services related to mandated consultation and/or related services (e.g., PRO, third-party payer, governmental, legislative, or regulatory requirement) may be identified by adding the modifier 32 to the basic procedure.

Using the Modifier Correctly
- Modifier 32 is used when the physician is aware of third-party involvement regarding mandated services.
- Modifier 32 is considered informational and, when used, many insurers allow 100 percent reimbursement without a deductible or copay. However, modifier 32 has no effect on Medicare payment.

Incorrect Use of the Modifier
- Lack of understanding as to the intent of this modifier may lead to inappropriate assignment. Do not use this modifier when a patient or family member requests a second opinion from another physician.

Coding Tips
- Use modifier 32 to indicate services related to mandated procedures.
- CPT codes for use with modifier 32 are 99201–99499, 00100–01999, 10021–69990, 70010–79999, 80048–89399, and 90281–99600 unless limited by the payer.

Clinical Example
A newborn infant is diagnosed with a congenital heart defect that requires immediate surgery. The parents refuse the surgery based on religious beliefs. A court order is issued requiring the surgery, overriding the parents' religious convictions because without the surgery the patient would probably not survive.

The anesthesia code is submitted with modifier 32.

47   ANESTHESIA BY SURGEON

Regional or general anesthesia provided by the surgeon may be reported by adding the modifier 47 to the basic service. (This does not include local anesthesia.) **Note:** Modifier 47 would not be used as a modifier for the anesthesia procedures 00100–01999.

Special Note
This modifier is noted in this section for clarification purposes only. It should be reported by the surgeon performing the procedure and is appended to the CPT code representing the service. It is not to be reported by the anesthesiologist providing anesthesia services and is not appended to the anesthesia CPT codes 00100–01999. See the section titled, "Surgery" for a detailed explanation.

KEY POINT

Do not use modifier 47 (anesthesia by surgeon) with the anesthesia procedure codes 00100–01999. This modifier is reserved for use by the operating surgeon and should be appended to the surgeon's basic procedure code for the administration of regional or general anesthesia (local anesthesia is excluded).

51   Multiple Procedures

When multiple procedures other than evaluation and management services, are performed at the same session by the same provider, the primary procedure or service may be reported as listed. The additional procedure(s) or service(s) may be identified by appending the modifier 51 to the additional procedure or service code(s). **Note:** This modifier should not be appended to designated add-on codes.

Using the Modifier Correctly

- Modifier 51 is used when more than one surgical service is performed by the same physician on the same patient at the same session.
- Append modifier 51 to codes for the nonanesthesia multiple procedures performed by the anesthesiologist on the same day as the anesthesia (e.g., if in addition to the procedure a Swan-Ganz catheter [93503] and an arterial line were inserted [e.g., 36625]). Append modifier 51 to the code for the second procedure (e.g., 93503, 36620-51).
- The 51 modifier is used when separate and multiple anesthesia codes are used to report secondary procedures. If the same anesthesia code applies to two or more of the surgical procedures, enter the anesthesia code with modifier 51 and the number of surgeries to which the modified CPT code applies in the units field of the CMS-1500 claim form. The reporting protocol may vary according to third-party payers.

Incorrect Use of the Modifier

- Use of modifier 51 when the multiple services are performed by different physicians.
- When coding multiple surgeries, don't confuse them with procedures that are components of or incidental to a primary procedure. The intraoperative services, incidental surgeries or components of more major surgeries are not separately billable (e.g., laparotomy, lysis of adhesions, omentectomies).
- Using the 51 modifier in institutions where the anesthesiologist performs an anesthesia procedure and placement of a Swan-Ganz catheter, but in which no other procedures are performed by the anesthesiologist.

Coding Tips

- Modifier 51 is used when multiple procedures are performed on the same day and at the same session by the same provider. It will be necessary to check with your third-party payers to determine whether the anesthesia codes or the surgical codes should be used.
- If the anesthesiologist performs multiple procedures (i.e., catheter placement for central venous line and emergency intubation) on the same day, the multiple surgery payment rules apply (i.e., 100 percent of the fee for the highest valued procedure and 50 percent of the fee for the second procedure).
- Documentation should be made in the patient's record and should include the patient's history, extenuating circumstances (i.e., level of pain, interruption of activities of daily living), specific diagnosis codes, drugs injected, the specific site of each injection, dosage of the drug, the medical necessity for giving the injection and the expected outcome of the treatment.
- It may be necessary to use codes 99100, 99116, 99135, and 99140 to indicate qualifying circumstances. Some Medicaid carriers and commercial payers will approve additional payment for these codes. Medicare bundles payment for these circumstances into the anesthesia allowable.

Quick Tip

According to CMS's national policy (found in the *Medicare Carriers Manual*, (or CMS Web-based manual, pub 100-4, chapter12, section 50) sections 8312, 15018A, 15018E, and 15018G describing indications/limitations of coverage), CPT codes 00100–01999 qualify for reimbursement when the following types of anesthesia are administered:

- Inhalation
- Regional:
  −spinal (low spinal, saddle block)
  −epidural (caudal)
  −nerve block (retrobulbar, brachial plexus block, etc.)
  −field block
- Intravenous
- Rectal

- CPT codes for use with modifier 51 are 00100–01999, 10021–69990, 70010–79999, and 90281–99600, when appropriate unless limited by the payer.

Clinical Example
A 90-year-old woman, in good health except for severe osteoporosis, fell in her home sustaining multiple injuries. As a result, an open treatment of a femoral neck fracture (27236) and a closed treatment of a supercondylar humeral fracture, without manipulation, (24530) were carried out at different times during the day. The anesthesia code for the second procedure would be billed with the 51 modifier. In addition, anesthesia CPT code 99100, anesthesia, for patient of extreme age under one year and over 70, is reported on the claim. Code 99100 is an add-on code and must always be reported with the code representing the primary procedure(s).

53 Discontinued Procedure

Under certain circumstances, the physician may elect to terminate a surgical or diagnostic procedure. Due to extenuating circumstances or those that threaten the well being of the patient, it may be necessary to indicate that a surgical or diagnostic procedure was started but discontinued. This circumstance may be reported by adding the modifier 53 to the code reported by the physician for the discontinued procedure. **Note:** This modifier is not used to report the elective cancellation of a procedure prior to the patient's anesthesia induction and/or surgical preparation in the operating suite. For outpatient hospital/ambulatory surgery center (ASC) reporting of a previously scheduled procedure/service that is partially reduced or cancelled as a result of extenuating circumstances, or for those that threaten the well being of the patient prior to or after administration of anesthesia, see modifiers 73 and 74.

Using the Modifier Correctly
- Modifier 53 is used when a procedure was actually started but had to be discontinued before completion. For example, a cardiac catheterization was discontinued when the catheter could not be advanced into the heart and was withdrawn without obtaining any diagnostic data. To continue would have put this patient at risk. The claim should be accompanied by the operative/procedure report so that a determination of the work involved can be made for pricing purposes.
- When the procedure was discontinued after anesthesia was induced, report the discontinued procedure using the appropriate CPT code with modifier 53.

Incorrect Use of the Modifier
- Using modifier 53 to report the elective cancellation of a procedure prior to the patient's anesthesia induction and/or surgical preparation in the operative suite.
- Using modifier 53 when a procedure is prematurely terminated, prior to the induction of anesthesia. The correct modifier to report these services is modifier 52.

Coding Tips
- Modifier 53 is used when, under extenuating circumstances or those that threaten the well-being of the patient, the physician elects to terminate a surgical or diagnostic procedure following the administration of anesthesia.

Hospital ASC and Outpatient Coders
Modifier 53 is not applicable in hospital ASC or hospital outpatient facilities in accordance with CPT's modifiers approved for ASC outpatient hospital use.

- For aborted or discontinued procedures, the appropriate ICD-9-CM diagnosis code (V64.1, V64.2, or V64.3) is reported as a secondary code. Follow individual third-party payers guidelines, as some payers and managed care organizations do not accept V codes.
- CPT codes for use with modifier 53 are 00100–01999, 10021–69990, 70010–79999, 80048–89399, and 90780–99600 unless limited by the payer.

Clinical Example

A 28-year-old male is admitted for drainage of a retropharyngeal abscess. The abscess was noted after a bout of acute tonsillitis and was caused by B-hemolytic streptococcus. There is marked asymmetry between the tonsillar fossae being displaced inferiorly and medially on the involved side.

The operative steps will involve incision and drainage in the upper outer quadrant or the most prominent portion of the abscess.

The anesthesiologist prepares the patient for surgery and induces anesthesia. As the surgeon prepares to make the incision, the patient is noted to have frequent episodes of premature ventricular contractions (PVCs) on the cardiac monitor. The surgeon feels it necessary to terminate the procedure due to patient risk and to obtain an opinion from a cardiologist.

The appropriate anesthesia code is submitted with the modifier 53, as well as HCPCS Level II modifier AA.

59 Distinct Procedural Service

Under certain circumstances, the physician may need to indicate that a procedure or service was distinct or independent from other services performed on the same day. Modifier 59 is used to identify procedures/services that are not normally reported together, but are appropriate under the circumstances. This may represent a different session or patient encounter, different procedure or surgery, different site or organ system, separate incision/excision, separate lesion, or separate injury (or area of injury in extensive injuries) not ordinarily encountered or performed on the same day by the same physician. However, when another already established modifier is appropriate it should be used rather than modifier 59. Only if no more descriptive modifier is available, and the use of modifier 59 best explains the circumstances, should modifier 59 be used.

Using the Modifier Correctly

- Use modifier 59 when a billing a combination of codes that would normally not be billed together. This modifier indicates that the ordinarily bundled code represents a service done at a different anatomic site or at a different session on the same date. This may represent:
  —different session or patient encounter
  —different procedure or service/same day
  —different site or organ system (e.g., a skin graft and an allograft in different locations)
  —separate incision/excision
  —separate lesion (e.g., a biopsy of skin on the neck is performed at the same session as an excision of a 1.0 cm benign lesion of the face)

 Key Point

Do not bill Medicare more than once for the same anesthesia procedure code for the same patient on the same date of service unless the anesthesia services were rendered at different operative sessions. In these cases (if applicable), report the additional anesthesia services with modifier 59 to identify that the procedures are separate and distinct. If two or more identical anesthesia codes are billed on the same day for the same patient without the appropriate modifier, Medicare will consider the service with the highest DUT (day/unit/time) or NOS (number of services) for reimbursement, and Medicare will deny the other service(s).

Ingenix Coding Lab: Understanding Modifiers

- Use modifier 59 only on the procedure designated as the distinct procedural service. The physician needs to document that a procedure or service was distinct or separate from other services performed on the same day.
- Ensure the medical record documentation is clear as to the separate distinct procedure before appending modifier 59 to a code. This modifier allows the code to bypass edits so appropriate documentation must be present in the record. **Note:** Medicare uses Correct Coding Initiative (CCI) screens when editing claims for possible unbundling. Under CCI screens, specific codes are identified that should not be billed together.
- Use modifier 59 only if another modifier does not describe the situation more accurately.

Incorrect Use of the Modifier

- Appending modifier 59 with E/M codes.
- Reporting modifier 59 with radiation therapy management codes.
- Using modifier 59 when another modifier is more appropriate such as 24, 25, 78, or 79.

Coding Tips

- Modifier 59 is used to indicate that a procedure or service was distinct or independent from other services performed on the same day.
- All other possible modifier choices should be reviewed before using modifier 59. It is typically the modifier of last choice.
- If there is not a more descriptive modifier available and the use of modifier 59 best explains the circumstance, then report the service with modifier 59.
- The 59 modifier is used when the physician performs an injection of a diagnostic, therapeutic or antispasmodic substance (including narcotics), CPT codes 62310–62319. These codes could be used on the day of surgery by the anesthesiologist if the injection was not performed by the anesthesiologist as the type of anesthesia provided for the surgery. If the injection was performed by the anesthesiologist following surgery (same day) for postoperative pain relief, the 59 modifier indicates this circumstance. The procedure must be well documented in the medical record and medical necessity must be clearly recorded.
- If 62311 or 62319 are performed on the same day as an anesthesia service, append modifier 59 when the procedure is performed as a separate service from the anesthesia service. If the epidural catheter is placed on a different date from the surgery, then modifier 59 would not be necessary.
- Additional spine and spinal cord injection procedures, beyond one, may be allowed when the codes are billed with modifier 59. Documentation must be made in the patient's chart that adequately explains the patient's history and the extenuating circumstances.
- CPT codes for use with modifier 59 are 00100–01999, 10021–69990, 70010–79999, 80048–89399, and 90281–99600, when appropriate unless limited by the payer.
- Ventilation management/pulmonary services are separately reimbursable if performed after transfer out of postanesthesia recovery to a hospital unit/ICU. The anesthesiologist would append modifier 59 to the procedure code billed (codes 94656 or 94660–94662).

> ✓ **QUICK TIP**
>
> There are revised criteria and documentation requirements for medical direction services furnished on or after January 1, 1999. Medical direction is covered by Medicare when the following criteria are met and the physician:
>
> - Performs a preanesthesia exam/evaluation
> - Prescribes a plan for the patient's anesthesia
> - Personally participates in the most demanding procedures of the anesthesia plan, including induction and emergence if appropriate
> - Ensures that any procedures in the anesthesia plan, not personally performed, are done by a qualified anesthetist
> - Monitors the course of anesthesia administration at intervals
> - Remains physically present and available for immediate diagnosis and treatment of emergencies
> - Provides the indicated postanesthesia care
>
> All the above activities must be documented in the patient's medical record.

Clinical Examples

Example #1:
A 55-year-old female presents for a bladder repair (MMK) for ureteral prolapse and stress incontinence. The physician makes a horizontal incision in the abdomen just above the symphysis pubis. The bladder is suspended by placing sutures through the tissue surrounding the urethra and into the vaginal wall. The urethra is moved forward due to the tissues being sutured and pulled tightly up to the symphysis pubis. The patient is taken to recovery in good condition. However, several hours later, the patient's pain is intolerable and her gynecologist requests that a postoperative epidural be given by the anesthesiologist.

The procedure code for the placement of the postoperative epidural with modifier 59 is submitted. Documentation in the medical record must be present supporting this service and reason for it.

Example #2:
A patient undergoes arthroscopic knee surgery with general anesthesia. The anesthesiologist bills for CPT code 01382 for "anesthesia for arthroscopic procedures of knee joint." Subsequent to the procedure, on the same day, postoperative pain is sufficient to warrant an epidural catheter. CPT code 62311-59 would be billed indicating that this was a separate service from the anesthesia service.

Other Anesthesia Modifiers

The physical status modifiers, P1 through P6, signify six levels of patient-specific health factors and are to be reported with an anesthesia procedure code (00100–01999).

- P1   A normal healthy patient
- P2   A patient with mild systemic disease
- P3   A patient with severe systemic disease
- P4   A patient with severe systemic disease that is a constant threat to life
- P5   A moribund patient that is not expected to survive without the operation
- P6   A declared brain-dead patient whose organs are being removed for donor purposes

Because of the inconsistency between Medicare carriers and state Medicaid programs, HCPCS Level III or local modifiers are not detailed in this publication.

 KEY POINT

Anesthesia services should be reported with physical status modifiers consistent with the American Society of Anesthesiologists ranking of the patient's physical status. The physician should document the status as P1–P6 in the anesthesia record. See other anesthesia modifiers at the end of this section.

Chapter 3: Surgery

22 UNUSUAL PROCEDURAL SERVICES

When the service(s) provided is greater than that usually required for the listed procedure, it may be identified by adding modifier 22 to the usual procedure number. A report may also be appropriate.

Using the Modifier Correctly

- The 22 modifier is appended to the basic CPT procedure code when the service(s) provided is greater than usually required for the listed procedure. Use of modifier 22 allows the claim to undergo individual consideration.
- Modifier 22 is used to identify an increment of work that is infrequently encountered with a particular procedure and is not described by another code.
- The frequent reporting of modifier 22 has prompted many carriers to simply ignore it. When using modifier 22, the claim must be accompanied by documentation and a cover letter explaining the unusual circumstances. Documentation includes, but is not limited to, descriptive statements identifying the unusual circumstances, operative reports (state the usual time for performing the procedure and the prolonged time due to complication, if appropriate), pathology reports, progress notes, office notes, etc. Language that indicates unusual circumstances would be difficulty, increased risk, extended, hemorrhage, blood loss over 600cc, unusual findings, etc. If slight extension of the procedure was necessary (a procedure extended by 15–20 minutes) or, for example, routine lysis of adhesions was performed, these scenarios do not validate the use of the modifier 22.
- Surgical procedures that require additional physician work due to complications or medical emergencies may warrant the use of modifier 22 after the surgical procedure code.
- Modifier 22 is applied to any code of a multiple procedure claim, regardless of whether that code is the primary or secondary procedure. In these instances, the Medicare carrier first applies the multiple surgery reduction rules (e.g., 100 percent, 50 percent, 50 percent, 50 percent, 50 percent). Then, a decision is made as to whether or not payment consideration for modifier 22 (unusual circumstances) is in order. For example, if the fee schedule amounts for procedures A, B, and C are $1000, $500, and $250 respectively, and a modifier 22 is submitted with procedure B, the carrier would apply the multiple surgery payment reduction rule first (major procedure 100 percent of the Medicare fee schedule) and reduce the procedure B (second surgical procedure) fee schedule amount from $500 to $250. The carrier would then decide whether or not to pay an additional amount above the $250 based on the documentation submitted with the claim for unusual procedural services, as designated by modifier 22.

Incorrect Use of the Modifier

- Appending this modifier to a surgical code without documentation in the medical record of an unusual occurrence. Because of its overuse, many payers do not acknowledge this modifier.
- Using this modifier on a routine basis; to do so would most certainly cause scrutiny of submitted claims and may result in an audit.

QUICK TIP

Hospital ASC and Outpatient Coders
Modifier 22 is not applicable in hospital ASC or hospital outpatient facilities in accordance with CPT's modifiers approved for ambulatory surgery center (ASC) outpatient hospital use.

- Using modifier 22 to indicate that the procedure was performed by a specialist, specialty designation does not warrant use of the 22 modifier.

Coding Tips

- Using modifier 22 identifies the service as one requiring individual consideration and manual review.
- Overuse of the modifier 22 could trigger a carrier audit. Carriers monitor the use of this modifier very carefully. Make sure that the 22 modifier is used only when sufficient documentation is present in the medical record.
- A Medicare claim submitted with the 22 modifier is forwarded to the carrier medical review staff for review and pricing. With sufficient documentation of medical necessity, increased payment may result.
- Do not bombard the Medicare carrier or other third-party payer with unnecessary documentation. All attachments to the claim for justification of the unusual services should explain the unusual circumstances in a concise, clear manner. The information for the justification of unusual services should be easy to locate within the attached documentation. Highlight this information, if necessary, to facilitate the medical reviewer's access to the pertinent supporting data.
- Modifier 22 is used on all procedure codes with a Medicare global period of zero, 10, or 90 days when unusual circumstances warrant consideration of payment in excess of the fee schedule allowance. This includes services that have a global period but are not surgical services.
- For a nonparticipating physician, the limiting charge provisions (see next bullet) apply to services that are billed with the modifier 22 and to all claims submitted to Medicare as a secondary payer, if the services billed are those on the physician fee schedule and subject to charge limits. In all cases the limiting charge cannot exceed a percentage of the allowable amount. This is the case even in instances where the allowance amount will not be known until the claim is individually priced.
- A claim with modifier 22 will be processed on a by-report basis and will cause the claim processing to be delayed. In these cases Medicare will consider the unusual nature of the service and, if they believe a charge above the fee schedule is justified, will approve an amount that recognizes the additional services. This in effect becomes a higher-than-usual fee schedule amount for the service. The approved amount (or higher fee schedule amount) is the basis of the limiting charge calculation for modifier 22 services. Therefore, if the billed amount exceeds Medicare's approved amount by more than 15 percent, make an adjustment or a refund to the patient in order to meet the limiting charge requirements of the law. Because the exact limiting charge on these cases is not known until an allowable amount decision is made, Medicare would not consider these cases as knowing or willful violations, provided the physician made the appropriate adjustments or refunds.
- CPT codes for use with modifier 22 are 00100–01999, 10021–69990, 70010–79999, 80048–89399, and 90281–99600 unless limited by the payer.

Clinical Example

The patient is a 3-year-old female brought to the emergency department (ED) by her mother after stepping on glass while playing outside. There is a piece of glass in her right foot as well as splinters of glass in both feet. The child is crying constantly and cannot be comforted. X-rays reveal a questionable, small radiopaque foreign body (FB) in the child's right foot. The patient is papoosed. Plain xylocaine is used as a

KEY POINT

Claims submitted to Medicare, Medicaid, and other third-party payers containing modifier 22 for unusual procedural services that do not have attached supporting documentation that demonstrates the unusual distinction of the services will generally be processed as if the procedure codes were not appended with the modifier. Some third-party payers might suspend the claims and request additional information, but this is the exception rather than the rule.

local anesthetic. The foot is incised with removal of a large piece of glass; this FB is deep and removal is complicated with bleeders encountered and cauterized. The removal of the glass splinters from the sites on both feet is time consuming and tedious. This procedure is significantly prolonged due to the multiple slivers of glass, dirt, and gravel in the wounds requiring partial skin thickness debridement and cleansing. What would normally take 40–45 minutes to complete actually has taken two hours. The patient is discharged home with her mother with a prescription for an analgesic and an antibiotic. She is to follow up with her pediatrician.

Submit CPT codes: 28193-22, 11040-59.

Note: The 59 modifier may be necessary to pass the initial payer edits, as the debridement may be considered part of the foreign body removal when it was on a different site.

26 PROFESSIONAL COMPONENT

Certain procedures are a combination of a physician component and a technical component. When the physician component is reported separately, the service may be identified by adding the modifier 26 to the usual procedure number.

Using the Modifier Correctly
- Modifier 26 is appended to the procedure code to report only the professional component.
- Modifier 26 is used in those instances in which a physician is providing the interpretation of the diagnostic test/study performed. The interpretation of the diagnostic test/study has to be separate, distinct, written and signed.

Incorrect Use of the Modifier
- Using modifiers 26 and TC for technical component (except for purchased diagnostic tests) when a diagnostic test or radiology service is performed globally (both components are performed by the same provider). When a global service is performed, the code representing the complete service should be reported without modifiers. The payment for the global service will reflect the allowances for both components. (For more information on HCPCS Level II modifier TC, see section "HCPCS Modifiers A-V.")
- Using the 26 modifier for a re-read of results of an interpretation initially provided by another physician.
- Using both modifier 26 indicating that only the professional portion of the service was provided and modifier 52 for reduced services. It is not necessary to use 52 because the professional component modifier already indicates that only a portion of the complete service was performed.

Coding Tips
- Certain procedures are a combination of a physician component and a technical component. To report the physician component separately, add modifier 26 to the procedure code.
- In order to use the professional component modifier 26, the provider must prepare a written report that includes findings, relevant clinical issues and, if appropriate, comparative data. This report must be available if requested by the carrier. A review of the diagnostic procedure findings, without a written report similar to that which would be prepared by a specialist in the field, does not meet the conditions for modifier use. The review of the findings, usually docu-

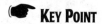

KEY POINT

There are certain procedure codes that describe and represent only the professional component portion of a procedure or service. These codes are stand-alone procedure or service codes, identifying the physician's or provider's professional efforts. In most cases, there are other procedure or service codes that identify the technical component only, and codes that represent both the professional and technical components as complete procedures or services called global service codes. It is not necessary to report modifier 26 with codes that aptly describe and represent only the professional component of a procedure or service.

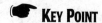

KEY POINT

In order to use a PC modifier 26, the provider must prepare a written report that includes findings, relevant clinical issues, and if appropriate, comparative data.

mented in the medical record or on a machine-generated report as "fx-tibia" or "EKG-WNL" with inverted Q-waves on lead II" does not suffice as a separately identifiable report, and is not eligible for payment. These types of procedural review notes should be bundled into any E/M code billed for that date. If a postpayment review of the medical record reveals that no separate, written interpretive report exists, overpayment recoveries may be sought.

- CPT codes for use with modifier 26 are 10021–69990, 70010–79999, 80048–89399, and 90281–99600 unless limited by the payer.

Clinical Examples

Example #1:
A complex cystometrogram is performed by a urologist and a certified technician in a hospital outpatient setting.

Submit code 51726-26. When the physician only interprets the results (or only operates the equipment), a professional component modifier 26 should be used to identify the physician's services.

Example #2:
The patient presents to the hospital urology outpatient clinic for a penile plethysmography due to priapism. The physician is present during the procedure and interprets the results.

Submit CPT code 54240-26.

Example #3:
The patient receives a urodynamic studies including a simple cystometrogram (CMG), a simple uroflowmetry and an electromyography (EMG) of the urethral sphincter performed at the hospital as outpatient procedures. The physician is present and performs the professional components of these procedures.

Submit codes 51784-26, 51725-51-26, and 51736-51-26.

32   MANDATED SERVICES

Services related to mandated consultation and/or related services (e.g., QIO, third-party payer, governmental, legislative, or regulatory requirement) may be identified by adding the modifier 32 to the basic procedure.

Using the Modifier Correctly

- Modifier 32 is used when the physician is aware of third-party involvement regarding mandated services.
- Documentation must support the use of modifier 32 for a mandated service and it must support medical necessity. Who and why must be clearly written in the medical record.
- Modifier 32 is considered informational and, when used, many insurers allow 100 percent reimbursement without a deductible or copay. However, modifier 32 has no effect on Medicare payment.

Incorrect Use of the Modifier

- Lack of understanding as to the intent of this modifier may lead to inappropriate assignment. Do not use this modifier when a patient or family member requests a second opinion.

Coding Tips
- Modifier 32 is used to indicate mandated evaluation and management services and/or procedures. Though infrequently reported with surgery codes, it is a valid modifier for surgical procedures.
- CPT codes for use with modifier 32 are 99201–99499, 00100–01999, 70010–79999, 80048–89399, and 90281–99600 unless limited by the payer.

Clinical Examples

Example #1:
A 38-year-old female, on fertility drugs, is now pregnant with eight known fetuses confirmed by ultrasound. This is her first pregnancy. The obstetrician feels a fetus reduction is necessary for the survival of the mother and fetuses. The patient refuses the multifetal pregnancy reduction (MPR) procedure and the physician requests the courts to make a decision. The court rules in favor of the physician and the surgery would be coded 59866-32.

47   Anesthesia By Surgeon

Regional or general anesthesia provided by the surgeon may be reported by adding the modifier 47 to the basic service. (This does not include local anesthesia.) **Note:** Modifier 47 or 09947 would not be used as a modifier for the anesthesia procedures 00100–01999.

Using the Modifier Correctly
- Modifier 47 is used when the anesthesia is administered by the operating physician. It denotes the use of regional or general anesthesia.

Incorrect Use of the Modifier
- Use of the modifier by the anesthesiologist
- Attaching the modifier to the anesthesia codes (00100–01999)
- Using the modifier 47 to bill for payment of local anesthesia a surgeon has administered.
- Reporting this modifier to Medicare (and many state Medicaid programs) with the CPT procedure code when the surgeon administers the regional or general anesthesia. This service is not covered by these programs.

Coding Tips
- Add modifier 47 to the basic service for regional or general anesthesia provided by the surgeon (this does not include local anesthesia), except for Medicare and many state Medicaid claims. See the Medicare alert on this page for a full explanation.
- Do not use modifier 47 on anesthesia procedure codes 00100–01999.
- CPT codes for use with modifier 47 are 10021–69990 unless limited by the payer.

Clinical Example
A surgeon performs a carpal tunnel release under a regional nerve block, which is personally administered by the surgeon.

Submit CPT code 64721-47 (regional nerve block performed by the surgeon). The addition of the 47 modifier tells the third-party payer the surgeon performed the anesthesia.

Key Point

Modifier 47 is appropriately used to report regional or general anesthesia (but not local anesthesia) provided by the physician performing the procedure or service requiring the anesthetic. This service, however, is not covered by Medicare and many state Medicaid programs. Commercial plans and managed care organizations, however, may cover this additional service.

50 BILATERAL PROCEDURE

Unless otherwise identified in the listings, bilateral procedures that are performed at the same operative session should be identified by adding the modifier 50 to the appropriate five-digit code.

Using the Modifier Correctly

- The 50 modifier is used only when the exact same service/code is reported for each bilateral anatomical site.
- For Medicare claims, report the bilateral procedures with one procedure code appended with modifier 50. This should appear on the CMS-1500 claim form as one-line item, with a unit number of one. However, many Medicare carriers will also accept bilateral procedures reported as two-line items with the right (RT) and left (LT) HCPCS Level II modifiers appended to the respective procedure codes.
- When the 50 modifier is reported, Medicare payment for surgical procedures is reimbursed at 150 percent of the fee schedule, taking into consideration any multiple surgery adjustments.
- Lacrimal punctum plugs are used to close the puncta located at the inner corners of the eyes. Procedure code 68761 identifies the closure of a single punctum. If the procedure is performed on both eyes, report 68761-50. In situations where two puncta are treated in the same eye, submit code 68761-76 and RT or LT. In situations where two puncta are treated in different eyes, submit code 68761-RT or LT on the first line, and 68761 RT or LT and 76 on the second line. If four puncta are closed, the physician should bill 68761-50 on the first line and 68761-76-50 on the next line. A written report (operative note) may be required with the claim.

Incorrect Use of the Modifier

- Using the 50 modifier on a bilateral procedure performed on different areas of the right and left sides of the body. This only applies to identical anatomical sites that have right and left sides, aspects or organs (e.g., arms, legs, eyes, hips, etc.). For example, modifier 50 would not be reported for a lesion removal performed on the right arm and a lesion removal performed on the left arm. This situation would not qualify as bilateral.
- Appending modifier 50 to a procedure that is identified in its description as a bilateral service. Report this procedure on one line without the 50 modifier as the relative value for the procedure already includes services for both sides. For example, the description of CPT code 69210 is removal of impacted cerumen, one or both ears. The Medicare physician fee schedule database (MPFSDB) identifies procedures considered bilateral with an indicator of 2 in the bilateral surgery field.
- Using modifier 50 when reporting procedure codes that are primarily bilateral by definition (e.g., lengthening of hamstring tendon; multiple, bilateral).
- Attaching modifier 50 to CPT surgical procedures that contain the words one or both (e.g., 69210—removal of cerumen, one or both ears).
- Using the 50 modifier to report procedure code 52005 as a bilateral procedure, for Medicare claims. The definition of a bilateral procedure does not apply to code 52005 (cystourethroscopy) as the basic procedure is an examination of the bladder and urethra which are not paired organs. The work relative value units are assigned taking into account the fact that it may be necessary to examine and catheterize one or both ureters. According to the Medicare physician fee schedule database (MPFSDB) the bilateral surgery indicator is "0," which reads:

©2003 Ingenix, Inc.
CPT only ©2003 American Medical Association. All Rights Reserved.

"the bilateral adjustment is inappropriate for codes in this category (a) because of physiology or anatomy, or (b) because the code description specifically states that it is a unilateral procedure and there is an existing code for the bilateral procedure." However, according *to CPT Assistant*, October 2001 instructions allow modifier 50 on CPT code 52005.

- Reporting bilateral procedures to Medicare as two line items on the CMS-1500 claim form, appending modifier 50 to the second bilateral procedure code as is correctly done for many other third-party payers. See the following "Quick Tip."
- Using 50 if one horizontal muscle of the right eye is operated upon, and the superior oblique muscle of the left eye is operated upon as well. The individual ocular muscles are represented by different codes. These procedures are reported as 67311 and 67318. Append modifier RT to code 67311. List code 67318 with modifier LT on the claim form.

Coding Tips

- Bilateral procedures that are performed at the same operative session should be identified by the appropriate CPT code for the first procedure. Add the 50 modifier to the second (bilateral) procedure code for non-Medicare claims.
- Check the MPFSDB for an indicator that will show whether or not a 50 modifier can be appended to the procedure for Medicare claims.
- Do not append the 50 modifier when tonsillectomy and adenoidectomy, codes 42820–42836, are performed bilaterally. If the procedure is performed unilaterally, then the appropriate code would be reported with modifier 52.
- CPT code 30130, excision turbinate, partial or complete, any method, is considered a unilateral procedure. If performed on both sides of the nose, append the 50 modifier to the code to indicate that a bilateral procedure was performed.
- CPT codes for use with modifier 50 are 10021–69990, 70010–79999, and 90281–99600 unless limited by the payer.

Clinical Examples

Example #1:
A physician repairs bilateral reducible inguinal hernias on a four-year-old child. An incision is made in the groin area. The hernia sac is identified. The hernia sac is resected, opened and returned to the abdominal cavity in correct anatomical position. The sac is sutured at the base. The procedure is repeated on the contralateral side. The muscle and fascia are repaired. The groin incision is closed and the patient returned to recovery room in stable condition. CPT code 49500-50 is submitted.

Example #2:
A 68-year-old female Medicare patient undergoes a bilateral lumbar laminotomy with partial fasciotomy, foraminotomy, and excision of a herniated intervertebral disc, for nerve root decompression. A posterior midline incision is made, the ligamentum flavum is partially removed. The lamina is removed, fragments of the disks and facets are removed. When decompression is achieved, the graft is placed to protect the nerve root. The paravertebral muscles are repositioned and the tissue is closed in layers.

CPT code 63030-50 is submitted, reporting the primary procedure and the bilateral (second) procedure together with one-line item for this Medicare patient.

Quick Tip

Medicare guidelines for the use of modifier 50 differ from many third-party payers' accepted protocol. In part, the definition of modifier 50 found in the 2000 CPT manual reflects the Medicare perspective in this modifier's use for Medicare claims. The *Medicare Carriers Manual*, CAR3 4827.B (or CMS Web-based manual, pub 100–4, chapter 12 section 40.7) states, "If a procedure is not identified by its terminology as a bilateral procedure (or unilateral or bilateral), report the procedure with modifier 50. Report such procedures as a single line item."

For instance, if the bilateral otoplasty procedures cited in the previous quick tip example were performed on a Medicare patient, both procedures would be reported as follows:

69300-50   Otoplasty, protruding ear, with or without size reduction

The second, or bilateral, procedure is inherent in the one line-item by the 50 modifier being appended to the appropriate procedure code.

Note: Some Medicare carriers will also accept bilateral procedures reported as two-line items with the right (RT) and left (LT) HCPCS Level II modifiers appended to the respective procedure codes.

Ingenix Coding Lab: Understanding Modifiers

Example #3:

A 28-year-old patient being treated for several years by her gynecologist due to infertility, presents for laparoscopy with bilateral salpingostomy. The physician inserts two instruments into the vagina. A laparoscope is then inserted through the umbilicus and the pelvic organs are viewed. A new opening is made in both fallopian tubes where stricture of the lumen of each tube has occurred, secondary to infection, imflammation, or injury.

CPT code 58673-50 is submitted. The individual commercial payers can ascertain if the bilateral service is to be reported as a single line item with the 50 modifier, or a two-line item with the 50 placed on the second (bilateral) procedure code, as shown in this example of the CMS-1500 form.

51   MULTIPLE PROCEDURES

When multiple procedures, other than evaluation and management services, are performed at the same session by the same provider, the primary procedure or service may be reported as listed. The additional procedure(s) or service(s) may be identified by appending the modifier 51 to the additional procedure or service code(s). **Note:** This modifier should not be appended to designated add-on codes or codes with ⊘ modifier 51 exemption.

Using the Modifier Correctly

- Use modifier 51 to indicate that more than one surgical service was performed by the same physician on the same patient at the same session.

- When more than one classification of wound repairs is performed, use the 51 modifier.

- When coding a bronchoscopy and a laryngoscopy with tracheotomy tube change, append the 51 modifier on the second code.

- Use 51 for the delivery of twins. In the situation of a twin vaginal delivery, use CPT codes 59400 (twin A) and 59409-51 (twin B). If one twin was delivered vaginally and one twin cesarean, use CPT codes 59510 and 59409-51.

- Multiple surgeries are separate procedures performed by the same physician on the same patient at the same operative session. A multiple surgical payment reduction is applied by Medicare as the major surgery includes payment for patient preparation time and services. Report the major procedure without the 51 modifier and additional procedures with the 51 modifier. Medicare determines the major procedure based upon the highest Medicare fee schedule amount of the surgeries performed/reported. The major procedure is paid based on 100 percent of the fee schedule amount. Payment for the additional procedures is based on 50 percent of the Medicare fee schedule amount. Some surgical procedures are not subject to multiple surgery reduction guidelines.

- Report multiple surgeries on the same claim using the 51 modifier. Avoid fragmenting or unbundling a comprehensive service into its component parts and reporting each component as if it were a separate service. For example, the correct CPT code to report for upper gastrointestinal endoscopy with biopsy of stomach is CPT code 43239. Separating the service into two parts, and using, for instance, CPT code 43235 for the basic service of upper gastrointestinal endoscopy with CPT code 43600 for biopsy of stomach is inappropriate reporting of services.

- When more than five surgical procedures are billed on the same date, Medicare requires that modifier 51 be reported and documentation accompany the claim.

✓ **QUICK TIP**

Hospital and Outpatient Coders
Modifier 51 is not applicable in hospital ASC or hospital outpatient facilities in accordance with CPT modifiers approved for ASC outpatient hospital use.

©2003 Ingenix, Inc.
CPT only ©2003 American Medical Association. All Rights Reserved.

- Options may exist when reporting multiple procedures. For example, the medical record procedure note states "tenolysis for six flexors in the wrist." The description for CPT code 25295 is tenolysis, flexor or extensor tendon, forearm and/or wrist, single, each tendon. CPT code 25295 can be coded once, with the number 6 in the units column. However, it is also appropriate to list each code and use the modifier 51 on the all codes except the first. For the preferred method of coding, check with the third-party payer.
- Medicare has a special endoscopy policy. If the multiple endoscopic procedures are in the same related family, the 51 modifier is not applied and payment is based on the special endoscopic policy. If the multiple endoscopic procedures are in a different endoscopic family (unrelated) the modifier 51 would be placed on the secondary (unrelated) procedure.

Incorrect Use of the Modifier

- Using 51 on procedures that are considered components or incidental to a primary procedure. The intraoperative services, incidental surgeries, or components of more major surgeries are not separately billable (e.g., laparotomy, lysis of adhesions, omentectomies).
- Using 51 in instances in which two or more phyicians each perform distinctly different, unrelated surgeries on the same day/same patient (e.g., multiple trauma cases). Using modifier 51 only if one surgeon individually performs multiple surgeries.
- Reporting code 45334 with the 51 modifier to describe any control of iatrogenically caused bleeding if an endoscopic biopsy is performed in the sigmoid colon and the excision of the tissue specimen causes bleeding that is controlled endoscopically. Report only code 45334.
- Appending the modifier 51 to code 22851 when the fracture treatment, dislocation or arthrodesis is performed in addition to spinal instrumentation. Report the appropriate fracture treatment, dislocation or arthrodesis code separately without the 51 modifier in addition to code 22851.

Coding Tips

- When multiple procedures, other than E/M services, are performed on the same day or at the same session by the same provider, report the primary procedure or service and append the 51 modifier to the appropriate CPT code(s) for the additional service(s) or procedure(s).
- Do not use the 51 modifier with add-on codes. Add-on codes are procedures performed in addition to the main procedure. These codes represent procedures which cannot be performed alone. Examples of words to look for as clues to add-on procedures are, each additional, list in addition to, and second lesion.
- CPT codes for use with modifier 51 unless limited by the payer are 00100–01999, 10021–69990, 70010–79999, and 90281–99600, when appropriate.

Clinical Examples

Example #1:
A 20-year-old male is transported to the ED via ambulance for multiple lacerations after walking into a glass door. After the initial examination, the ED physician performs debridement and repair of the following lacerations:

- 2.6-cm scalp laceration, simple 12002
- 2.4-cm neck laceration, simple 12001
- 2.3-cm facial laceration, simple 12011

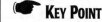 **KEY POINT**

The symbols: + and Ø are two symbols listed in the CPT manual. The + symbol is seen adjacent to CPT codes that represent "add-on" services, or services commonly carried out in addition to a primary procedure. These add-on codes are, therefore, not to be reported without first reporting the primary procedure code. The Ø symbol identifies CPT codes with which the -51 modifier, multiple procedures, should not be reported. For example, CPT code 17004 describes the destruction of benign or premalignant lesions, including local anesthesia, for 15 or more lesions. This code should not be reported with the 51 modifier as the destruction procedures for each of the 15 lesions are inherent in the code's description. Likewise, it should not be reported on the CMS-1500 claim form with a units quantity of 15, as only one unit correctly represents the service.

KEY POINT

When reporting wounds within the same classification and level, the lengths of each of the wounds repaired should be added together and reported under the CPT code designating the sum of those particular wound repair lengths. Classification is the grouping of like tissue types such as scalp, neck, external genitalia, trunk and extremities, and another such classification involves the face, ears, eyelids, nose, lips, and mucous membranes. The level of repair is classified as simple, intermediate, or complex. In clinical example #1, note that CPT code 12001 for the 2.4 cm laceration is not reported separately; it is combined with the length of the similarly classified wound described by CPT code 12002. These repairs are, therefore, reported only by the single CPT code 12002, representing a total wound repair length of 5.0 cm. This CPT code describes wound repair lengths ranging from 2.6 cm to 7.5 cm.

- 2.4-cm eyelid laceration, intermediate 12051
- 2.5-cm forearm laceration, complex 13120

The following CPT codes are submitted, following the CPT code book guidelines for repair (closure) of wounds. Note that the lengths of two of the wounds described, both being similar in classification, have been added together and are reported by one CPT code (12002).

- 13120
- 12051-51
- 12011-51
- 12002-51

Example #2:

The physician performs an excision of a benign lesion on the patient's face; the excision is 0.3 cm in diameter. At the same session, a biopsy is taken of the skin and subcutaneous tissue from a lesion on the patient's low back area.

CPT codes 11440 and 11100-51 are submitted.

(**Note:** Modifier 59 may be placed on CPT code 11100 to designate a separate site. Check with the payer about acceptance of modifier 59.)

Example #3:

A vertebral laminotomy is performed on two lumbar disks involving two interspaces. Arthrodesis of the two lumbar interspaces (anterior technique) is also done at the same operative session.

CPT codes 63030, 63035, 22558-51, and 22585 are submitted.

Codes 63035 and 22585 are considered add-on procedure codes and modifier 51 should not be used when these codes are reported.

Example #4:

The patient presents to the otorhinolaryngologist for a planned excision of a dermoid cyst from her nose, on the right side. During the preprocedure examination, the physician notes three polyps in the left nostril. The decision is made to excise these polyps at the same session as the cyst excision.

CPT codes 30124 and 30110-51 are submitted.

Example #5:

Resection is carried out of a fibrous histiocytoma of the upper arm (5 cm skin margins). The underlying biceps muscle is resected with an in-continuity axillary node dissection. The defect is reconstructed with a latissimus dorsi muscle flap to restore elbow flexion and a 250 sq cm STSG (split thickness skin graft).

Submit CPT codes 15734 (latissimus dorsi muscle flap), 38745-51 (axillary lymphadenectomy), 24077-51 (radical resection sarcoma of the arm), 15100-51 (STSG, first 100 sq cm), 15101 (STSG, next 100 sq cm) and 15101 (STSG, next 100 sq cm).

If the information is available, report the services according to the relative value unit (RVU) for commercial payers or resource based relative value system (RBRVS) for

Medicare claims rankings, reporting the heavier ranked services first. In this case, these services would be reported as follows:

- 15734
- 24077-51
- 38745-51
- 15100-51
- 15101
- 15101

Note that CPT code 15101 is not appended with modifier 51 because it is an add-on code. The double listing of this code might be alternatively submitted as a single line item with a units value of two, depending upon carrier preference.

52 REDUCED SERVICES

Under certain circumstances a service or procedure is partially reduced or eliminated at the physician's discretion. Under these circumstances the service provided can be identified by its usual procedure number and the addition of the modifier 52, signifying that the service is reduced. This provides a means of reporting reduced services without disturbing the identification of the basic service. **Note:** For hospital outpatient reporting of a previously scheduled procedure/service that is partially reduced or canceled as a result of extenuating circumstances or those that threaten the well-being of the patient prior to or after administration of anesthesia, see modifiers 73 and 74.

Using the Modifier Correctly
- Use modifier 52 for reporting services that were partially reduced or eliminated at the physician's election. Documentation should be present in the medical record explaining the circumstances surrounding the reduction in services.
- Modifier 52 is used to indicate that a procedure or service is being performed at a lesser level. A concise statement that describes how the service differs from the normal procedure must be included with the claim or in the appropriate field for electronic claims.

Incorrect Use of the Modifier
- Using modifier 52 for terminated procedures. This modifier is intended for procedures that accomplished some result, but less than expected for the procedure.

Coding Tips
- Modifier 52 is used to indicate that, under certain circumstances, a service or procedure is partially reduced or eliminated at the physician's discretion.
- The use of this modifier may affect payment, and reduction in payment may occur.
- The 52 modifier is for a reduced service and is not a modifier to be used in situations when the fee is reduced for a patient due to his or her inability to pay the full charge.
- CPT codes for use with modifier 52 (unless limited by the payer) are 99201–99499 (except for Medicare), 10021–69990, 70010–79999, 80048–89399, and 90281–99600 (except psychotherapy), when appropriate.

QUICK TIP

Hospital ASC and Outpatient Coders
Per Medicare, modifier 52, reduced service, is used in the hospital outpatient department to identify a procedure not requiring anesthesia (meaning general, regional, or local) that was terminated after the patient was prepared for the procedure (including any sedation). Reimbursement for modifier 52 procedures is 50 percent.

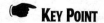

KEY POINT

The *Medicare Carriers Manual* states, in part, that when surgical procedures for which services performed are significantly less than usually required, [these services] may be billed with modifier 52. Surgical procedures reported with this modifier should include the following documentation:

- A concise statement about how the service or procedure differs from the usual
- The operative report

Clinical Example

A radical trachelectomy, with unilateral pelvic lymphadenectomy and para-aortic lymph node sampling biopsy, with removal of the left tube and ovary are performed for metastatic cervical cancer.

CPT code 57531-52 is submitted. The procedure was not completed per the CPT code description (bilateral pelvic lymphadenectomy) so modifier 52 would be appended to the procedure code.

53   DISCONTINUED PROCEDURE

Under certain circumstances, the physician may elect to terminate a surgical or diagnostic procedure. Due to extenuating circumstances or those that threaten the well-being of the patient, it may be necessary to indicate that a surgical or diagnostic procedure was started but discontinued. This circumstance may be reported by adding the modifier 53 to the code reported by the physician for the discontinued procedure. Note: This modifier is not used to report the elective cancellation of a procedure prior to the patient's anesthesia induction and/or surgical preparation in the operating suite. For outpatient hospital/ASC reporting of a previously scheduled procedure/service that is partially reduced or canceled as a result of extenuating circumstances or those that threaten the well-being of the patient prior to or after administration of anesthesia, see modifiers 73 and 74.

Using the Modifier Correctly
- Use modifier 53 when a procedure was actually started, but was discontinued before completion due to the patient's condition.
- If the procedure was discontinued after anesthesia was induced, report the aborted procedure using the appropriate CPT code with modifier 53.
- If a surgery is discontinued due to uncontrollable bleeding, hypotension, neurologic impairment, or situations that threaten the well-being of the patient, append modifier 53 to the surgical procedure code.
- The 53 modifier also applies to the physician's office. All procedures billed with the 53 modifier may require documentation to be submitted with the claim.

Incorrect Use of the Modifier
- Using modifier 53 to report the elective cancellation of a procedure prior to the patient's anesthesia induction and/or surgical preparation in the operative suite.
- Using modifier 53 when a procedure is prematurely terminated or reduced due to physician election, prior to the induction of anesthesia. The correct modifier to report these services is modifier 52.
- Using modifier 53 on an E/M code. Many insurance companies do not recognize the 53 modifier on this type of service. Check with individual payers for use of 53 on an E/M code.

Coding Tips
- Use modifier 53 when, under extenuating circumstances or those that threaten the well-being of the patient, the physician elects to terminate a surgical or diagnostic procedure. Use this modifier when it may be necessary to indicate that a surgical or diagnostic procedure was started but discontinued following the administration of anesthesia.

- For aborted or discontinued procedures, report the appropriate ICD-9-CM diagnosis code (V64.1, V64.2, or V64.3). Follow individual third-party payer guidelines, as some payers and managed care organizations do not accept V codes.
- CPT codes for use with modifier 53 are 00100–01999, 10040–69990, 70010–79999, 80048–89399, and 90281–99600 unless limited by the payer.

Clinical Examples

Example #1:
A surgical oncologist begins a radical pelvic exenteration on a patient that had been previously treated for ovarian cancer in past years. Now, she has once again, been diagnosed with cancer that is extensive and requires a radical pelvic exenteration. The surgeon begins dissection, but terminates the procedure when it becomes evident that the cancer was more widespread than expected.

Submit CPT code 51597-53. A report should be sent describing the reason for termination of the procedure.

Example #2:
Patient presents with multiple common bile duct calculi. She requires lithotripsy to remove the stones. Her diagnosis is choledocholithiasis. The stones are too large to pass through sphincterotomy. The patient is prepped for surgery. Nasobiliary drain is in place. No acute distress noted prior to procedure. Medications given are diazepam 15.0 mg IV, and meperidine 75.0 mg IV. Shortly after the procedure began, the patient's blood pressure was recorded at 140/70 and subsequently dropped to 100/50. The procedure was discontinued. The patient was treated for hypotension and observed postcancellation of the procedure.

CPT code 43265-53 is submitted. A report should be sent describing the reason for termination of the procedure.

Example #3:
Operative Report:

Preoperative Diagnosis: Cholelithiasis.

Postoperative Diagnosis: Same.

Operation Performed:

 1. Laparoscopic cholecystectomy.

 2. Lysis of adhesions.

Anesthesia: General endotracheal.

Estimated Blood Loss: Less than 200 cc.; COMPLICATIONS—Heart arrhythmia. DRAINS: None. FLUIDS: 1400 cc of crystalloid, 2 liters of irrigation fluid.

Brief History of Present Illness: The patient is a gentlemen with a history of previous abdominal surgery secondary to small bowel obstruction from lymphoma and previous myocardial infarction two years ago. He underwent previous exploratory laparotomy and lysis of adhesions. He now presented with episodic right upper quadrant pain. Right upper quadrant ultrasound was performed and he was noted to

QUICK TIP

Hospital ASC and Outpatient Coders
Modifier 53 is not applicable in hospital ASC or hospital outpatient facilities in accordance with CPT's modifiers approved for ASC outpatient hospital use.

have cholelithiasis. After a thorough discussion regarding the benefits of laparoscopic surgery versus open cholecystectomy and discussion of risks such as bleeding, infection, intraperitoneal organ injury, and common duct injury, the patient was taken to the operating room and placed in supine position on the operating table. We elected to proceed with laparoscopic cholecystectomy under open technique and convert to open cholecystectomy if there were too many adhesions to allow for laparoscopic cholecystectomy.

Procedure: His abdomen was prepped with a Betadine prep and sterile surgical drapes were applied after the uneventful induction of general anesthesia.

We began the procedure by making a vertical incision superior to the umbilicus along the lines of his previous surgical scar with the #11 blade. The incision was approximately an inch in length and it was carried down to the fascial layers with the Metzenbaum scissors. We then grasped the fascia and proceeded through the fascial layers sharply with a #15 blade. We then were able to visualize the peritoneum and grasped it.

The peritoneum was entered into sharply as well. We then opened a small segment of the incision and were able to pass a finger into the peritoneal cavity. There were adhesions surrounding the incision; however, it appeared that we had entered into the peritoneal cavity in a small area that was free of any adhesions. We bluntly dissected circumferentially around the intended trocar site and were able to take down some small adhesions.

We then passed a trocar into the abdominal cavity and insufflated to 15 mm Hg of pressure. We then passed a camera in through the trocar and were able to maneuver this around more adhesions and visualize the right upper quadrant. We were able to clearly see the gallbladder beneath some adhesions and were able to visualize the right side of the falciform ligament as well as the right upper quadrant abdominal wall, where we intended to place 5-mm trocars.

At this point in the surgery, the patient developed a significant cardiac arrhythmia. The anesthesiologist worked to control the PVCs, but it was decided to discontinue the procedure due to potential risks to the patient.

CPT code 47562-53 is submitted with an operative report.

54   SURGICAL CARE ONLY

When one physician performs a surgical procedure and another provides preoperative and/or postoperative management, surgical services may be identified by adding the modifier 54 to the usual procedure.

Using the Modifier Correctly

- To use modifier 54 correctly, there must be an agreement for the transfer of care between physicians. Transfer of responsibility of care is determined by the date of the transfer order. If a transfer of care does not occur, the services of a physician, other than the surgeon, are reported by the appropriate E/M code or other code.

- Use the modifier 54 with surgical codes only. Submit the CPT procedure code with modifier 54 in item 24d of the CMS-1500 claim form if the physician performs the surgery but does not intend to provide any of the postoperative care. Report the date of the surgery in item 24a.
- If the surgeon relinquishes postoperative management to another physician, he/she need not submit additional documentation with the CMS-1500 claim form to demonstrate the date of the patient's transfer of care. As stated, the surgeon need only report the CPT procedure code(s) appended with modifier 54, and enter the date of surgery in item 24a of the claim form.
- Report modifiers 54 and 55 if the surgeon provides the surgery and a portion of the postoperative care. File the surgery code with the 54 modifier in item 24d, the date of the surgery in item 24a and a single unit in item 24a. On a separate line, list the surgery code with the 55 modifier in item 24d and the date of the surgery in item 24a, and indicate the relinquished date in item 19 of the CMS-1500 claim form or in the narrative portion of the HAO record for electronic claims.
- For each surgical CPT code, third-party payers have established a certain percentage for each of the three components (i.e., preoperative, intraoperative, and postoperative). If the split care modifiers (54, 55, 56) are used, these percentages help determine payment.

Incorrect Use of the Modifier
- Appending modifier 54 to a surgical procedure without a global surgery period (global surgery period equal to zero days).
- Using modifier 54 for a minor surgical service (global period zero or 10 days) performed in the ED for a patient who is referred back to his or her primary care physician or other non-ED provider for follow-up care.

Coding Tips
- At times, more than one physician will provide the services that are included in the global surgical package. This may occur when one physician performs the surgical procedure and a second physician provides the follow-up care. Add the 54 modifier to the procedure code if one physician does the surgery, but another physician provides the postoperative care.
- The modifier 54 is an indicator that multiple physicians are involved with the patient's surgical care. Each physician must report the service provided so that the correct payments will be made for each claim upon initial submission. For example, Medicare payment is limited to the same total amount as would have been paid if one physician provided all the care, regardless of the number of caregivers.
- Do not use a 54 if the physician is the covering physician (i.e., locum tenens) or part of the same group as the surgeon who performed the procedure and provided most of the postoperative care.
- CPT codes for use with modifier 54 are appropriate codes in the surgery section (10021–69990) and in the medicine section (90281–99600), unless limited by the third-party payer.

Clinical Examples

Example #1:
An orthopaedic surgeon treats a Medicare patient for an open tibial shaft fracture (27759). After several days of postoperative care and subsequent discharge, the remainder of the postoperative care was relinquished to the patient's attending

QUICK TIP

When one physician performs a patient's surgical service and another provides the postoperative management, an agreement for the transfer of care must be retained in the Medicare beneficiary's medical records. This agreement can be in the form of a letter, discharge summary, chart notation or other written documentation, but in any case, both the surgeon and the physician who intends to provide the postoperative management must have a copy of the agreement.

✓ QUICK TIP

Under federal guidelines, when a patient's surgical service and the subsequent postoperative care are rendered in different Medicare carrier localities, each service must be billed to the respective carrier servicing the different payment localities. Both modifier 54 and modifier 55 are appropriate for this kind of service reporting. For example, if a surgery is performed in carrier A's region but the postoperative management is provided in carrier B's locality, the surgery would be billed to carrier A with modifier 54 appended to the applicable CPT procedure codes, and the postoperative care would be billed to carrier B by reporting modifier 55 with the applicable CPT procedure codes. This guideline must be followed whether the services are performed by the same physician or physician group, or whether the services are performed by different physicians or physician groups.

✓ QUICK TIP

Hospital ASC and Outpatient Coders
Modifiers 54 and 55 are not applicable in hospital ASC or hospital outpatient facilities in accordance with CPT's modifiers approved for ASC outpatient hospital use.

---

physician. Submit CPT code 27759-54. The relinquished date must be noted in box 19 of the CMS-1500 claim form. In this situation, payment for the surgeon is 10 percent for preoperative service and 69 percent for intraoperative service; the total is 79 percent of the allowed amount for the surgical procedure. Medicare payment would subsequently be 80 percent of the allowable amount.

The patient's attending physician bills for the postoperative care by reporting the procedure code 27759 with modifier 55. The date of service is the same as the date of surgery; the place of service is the same as the place of service for the surgery. The acquired care date must be noted in box 19 of the CMS-1500 claim form or in the appropriate HAO field for electronic claims.

Payment for the attending doctor is 21 percent for postoperative care. Medicare payment is made at 80 percent of the allowable amount.

Example #2:
A cardiac surgeon performs an aortic valve replacement with stentless tissue valve (33410) and 30 days postoperative care. The patient had aortic valve stenosis.

The cardiac surgeon submits CPT code 33410-54 in item 24d, the date of the surgery in item 24a and a single unit in item 24a of the CMS-1500 claim form. Also indicate the relinquished date in item 19. If submitting the claim electronically, be sure that information from item 19 of the paper claim form is included in the appropriate HAO field so the payer will know the dates the physician relinquished postoperative care.

Example #3:
A neurosurgeon travels monthly to a rural location to perform surgery. On this trip he assessed a patient and performed brain surgery on the patient the next day. Follow-up care will be performed by a local surgeon.

The neurosurgeon performed a craniotomy for drainage of an intracranial abscess, infratentorial.

CPT code 61321-54 is submitted.

Example #4:
A patient presented to the ED with complaints of moderate left wrist pain after falling onto her outstretched hand after tripping on a high curb. X-rays confirmed an ulnar shaft fracture. The ED physician interpreted the wrist x-ray by written report, (73110, Complete, minimum of three views). The physician performed an evaluation and following the encounter, performed a closed treatment of the ulnar shaft fracture without manipulation.

CPT codes 25530-54 and 73110-26 are submitted.

55   POSTOPERATIVE MANAGEMENT ONLY

When one physician performs the postoperative management and another physician has performed the surgical procedure, the postoperative component may be identified by adding the modifier 55 to the usual procedure number.

Using the Modifier Correctly

- Use with surgical codes to indicate that only the postoperative care was performed (i.e., another physician performed the surgery). In this case, the postoperative component may be identified by adding the modifier 55 to the CPT procedure code.

- Modifier 55 is appended if a physician does not perform the surgery but does provide a portion of the postoperative care. List the assumed date in item 19 of the CMS-1500 claim form, the surgery code with the 55 modifier in item 24d, the date of service in item 24a, and one unit of service in item 24g. Electronic billing software should have a narrative data field for this information in the HAO record. Be sure that information from item 19 is included so the payer will know the date the physician assumed the postoperative care.

- Modifier 55 is used after discharge of the patient from the hospital and only after the patient has been seen for postoperative follow-up care.

- Providers need not state on the claim that care has been transferred. However, the *Medicare Carriers Manual*, sec. 4822.B, (or CMS Web-based manual, pub 100-4, chapter 12, section 40.1) states that the date on which care was relinquished or assumed, as applicable, must be shown on the claim.

- Where a transfer of postoperative care occurs, the receiving physician cannot bill for any part of the global services until he or she has provided at least one service (i.e., at least one postoperative visit has been rendered). Once the physician sees the patient, the physician may bill using the 55 modifier for the period beginning with the date on which he or she assumes care of the patient.

- For each surgical CPT code, third-party payers have established a certain percentage for each of the three components (i.e., preoperative, intraoperative and postoperative). If the split care modifiers (54, 55, 56) are used, these percentages help determine payment.

Incorrect Use of the Modifier

- Using modifier 55 on the surgery code if a physician other than the surgeon provides the inpatient postoperative care when the transfer of care occurs immediately after surgery. The physician other than the surgeon should bill these inpatient services using the subsequent hospital care codes (99231–99233).

Coding Tips

- At times, more than one physician will provide the services that are included in the global surgical package. This may occur when one physician performs the surgical procedure and a second physician provides the follow-up care. The 55 modifier is added to the procedure code if the physician provides the postoperative care, but another physician performed the surgical procedure.

- The 55 modifier is an indicator that multiple physicians are involved in the patient's surgical care. Each physician must report the service he or she provided so that the correct payments will be made for each claim upon submission. For example, Medicare payment is limited to the same total amount as would have been paid if one physician provided all the care, regardless of the number of caregivers. Payment for modifier 55 will be limited to the amount allotted for postoperative services only. In addition, when more than one physician is providing postoperative care, each physician would be paid based on the number of postoperative days that each cared for the patient (e.g., using a 90-day postoperative period, a 45/45-day split, 30/60-day split, 10/60/20-day split, etc.).

- The 55 modifier is appended to the surgery code only after the first postoperative visit is provided by the physician performing the postoperative management.

©2003 Ingenix, Inc.
CPT only ©2003 American Medical Association. All Rights Reserved.

- CPT codes for use with modifier 55 are appropriate codes in the surgery section (10040–69990) and in the medicine section (90281–99600), unless limited by the third-party payer unless limited by the payer.

Clinical Examples

Example #1:
An orthopaedic surgeon performs an open tibial shaft fracture (27759). The postoperative care for this patient will be relinquished to the patient's attending physician following discharge.

The attending physician should append the 55 modifier to code 27759 with the same date of the surgery, same place as the surgery and the assumed date of care reported in item 19 of the CMS-1500 claim form or the appropriate HAO narrative data field for electronic claims.

Example #2:
A second physician was involved in the postoperative care management (for 60 days of the 90-day global period) of a patient who had an aortic valve replacement with aortic annulus, enlargement noncoronary cusp, performed by a cardiac surgeon. The patient had aortic valve stenosis.

This physician would report, after initially seeing the patient, the surgery code (33411) appended with modifier 55. The date care was assumed must be noted in item 19 of the CMS-1500 claim form. However, the original surgery date should still be noted in item 24a of the CMS-1500 claim form (the fields for the From/To and Date(s) of Service).

Note: Both the surgeon's bill for the surgical care and the bill for the physician rendering postoperative care will contain the same date of service and the same surgical procedure code, with their respective services only differentiated by the use of the appropriate modifier (54 or 55).

56 PREOPERATIVE MANAGEMENT ONLY

When one physician performs the preoperative care and evaluation and another physician performs the surgical procedure, the preoperative component may be identified by adding the modifier 56 to the usual procedure number.

Using the Modifier Correctly

- The modifier 56 is added to the usual procedure number when one physician performs the preoperative care and evaluation but another physician performs the surgical procedure.
- For each surgical CPT code, third-party payers have established a certain percentage for each of the three components (i.e., preoperative, intraoperative and postoperative). If the split care modifiers (54, 55, 56) are used, these percentages help determine payment.
- Check with your Medicare carrier and other third-party payers for their instructions on the appropriate use of this modifier in your region. Modifier 56 is usually not used for Medicare claims. Payment for this modifier is included in the Medicare allowable for the surgery. If a different physician performs the preoperative service, use the appropriate E/M code. Follow your carrier's instructions for correct use of this modifier.

Hospital ASC and Outpatient Coders
Modifier 56 is not applicable in hospital ASC or hospital outpatient facilities in accordance with CPT's modifiers approved for ambulatory surgery center (ASC) outpatient hospital use.

Since the Medicare fee schedule amount for surgical procedures includes all component services that comprise the global surgical package (pre-, intra- and postoperative services), the sum of the Medicare approved amount for all of the physicians involved in the patient's care, even when fragmented into these components, will not exceed the typical global amount allowed if only one physician were to provide the entire surgical package. An exception to this policy occurs when the surgeon performs only the surgery and another physician—other than the surgeon—provides both the preoperative and postoperative inpatient care. This can result in a total payment to all involved physicians that is higher than the global surgery allowed amount.

Incorrect Use of the Modifier
- Adding modifier 56 to an E/M service code.

Coding Tips
- At times, more than one physician will provide the services that are included in the global surgical package. This may occur when one physician performs the surgical procedure and a second physician provides the follow-up care. Modifier 56 is applied to the code used for surgery if a physician provides only preoperative service.
- Modifier 56 is rarely utilized, and it should be used on surgical procedures only.
- CPT codes for use with modifier 56 are 10021–69990 unless limited by the payer.

Clinical Example
A patient living in a rural area is being seen for a preoperative work-up by her regular physician. She will be having a laparoscopic cholecystectomy for cholelithiasis the following morning by a general surgeon who travels to the rural area on a monthly basis. The preoperative care was done by the patient's internist and documented the day before the scheduled surgery.

CPT code 47562-56 is submitted.

58   STAGED OR RELATED PROCEDURE OR SERVICE BY THE SAME PHYSICIAN DURING THE POSTOPERATIVE PERIOD

The physician may need to indicate that the performance of a procedure or service during the postoperative period was: a) planned prospectively at the time of the original procedure (staged); b) more extensive than the original procedure; or c) for therapy following a diagnostic surgical procedure. This circumstance may be reported by adding the modifier 58 to the staged or related procedure. **Note:** This modifier is not used to report the treatment of a problem that requires a return to the operating room. See modifier 78.

Using the Modifier Correctly
- Use modifier 58 only when the second and/or related staged services are performed during the postoperative period of the original (first) procedure.
- A new postoperative period begins when the next procedure in the staged procedure series is billed. If more than one physician is involved in a staged procedure, each physician must submit the claim using the 58. These claims are subject to individual consideration and payment calculation is based on the percentage of the procedure each physician performs.
- In a case where a breast biopsy and mastectomy are performed on the same day, and the purpose of the biopsy is to determine if there is a malignancy before proceeding with the mastectomy because there has been no previous confirmation by biopsy, then report both the mastectomy and the biopsy. In this situation, report the biopsy with CPT modifier 58 to indicate that it is a staged procedure and CPT modifier 51 to indicate that it is a multiple procedure.
- Some injuries require multiple fracture debridement procedures in order to properly treat the fracture. There may be a situation calling for staged fracture debridement. These procedures often are performed on open fractures that have not yet been treated to accommodate the reduction of the bones. When performing a staged procedure, an initial fracture debridement may be performed

Hospital ASC and Outpatient Coders
Medicare's instructions for modifier 58 in hospital ASC or hospital outpatient facilities include in the definition procedures performed on the same calendar day.

Ingenix Coding Lab: Understanding Modifiers

for extension of the wound for exploration or excisional debridement and irrigation of all tissue layers. Repeat debridement may be required for a heavily contaminated wound or for other reasons. In these situations requiring repeat procedures following the initial debridement procedure, report the subsequent procedures with the modifier 58.

Incorrect Use of the Modifier

- Using modifier 58 to report the treatment of a problem that requires a return to the operating room. See modifier 78.
- Using modifier 58 for unrelated procedures performed during the postoperative period of the original (first) procedure or service. See modifier 79 for unrelated procedures performed by the same physician during the postoperative period, or modifiers 51 and 59, as appropriate, for multiple procedures and distinct procedural service for procedures performed by another physician during the postoperative period of the original surgery. (**Note:** For repeat procedures performed by another physician, see modifier 77.)

Coding Tips

- To report a staged or related procedure, add the modifier 58. Failure to use this modifier when appropriate may result in denial of the subsequent surgery claim.
- Do not use modifier 58 with CPT procedure codes that are described as one or more services (e.g., 67141, 67145, 67208, 67210, 67218, 67227, and 67228). These procedures in CPT are considered multiple sessions or are otherwise defined as including multiple services or events. The Medicare fee schedule RVU was established based on the sum of the total procedures; therefore, separate reimbursement may not be made for each segment of the procedure even if it is for one or more services.
- Do not use 58 with procedures that describe a subsequent stage such as 52614 or 17305–17307.
- CPT codes for use with modifier 58, unless limited by the payer, are 10021–69990, 70010–79999, and 90281–99600, as appropriate.

Clinical Examples

Example #1:
A breast biopsy (19120) is performed on one date. Then the patient is returned to the operating room within the postoperative period of the initial procedure for more extensive removal of breast tissue, such as, that required for a modified radical mastectomy for breast cancer.

CPT code 19240-58 is submitted.

Example #2:
Sternal debridement (21627) is performed for mediastinitis, and it is noted that a muscle flap repair (15734) will be needed in a few days of the sternal debridement to properly close the defect.

Submit CPT code 15734-58 since the muscle flap was planned at the time of the initial surgery.

Example #3:
An incisional prostate biopsy (55705) is done, and the specimen returns from the pathologist as "positive CA of the prostate." Within the 10-day follow up period of

QUICK TIP

Modifier 58 must be used for purposes of distinguishing surgical procedures performed by the original surgeon during the postoperative period of the original (first) procedure, within the constraints of the modifier's definition. These procedures cannot be repeat operations (unless the procedures are more extensive than the original procedure) and cannot be for the treatment of complications requiring a return trip to the operating room.

QUICK TIP

Modifier 58, among others, was the recent target of an investigation by various Medicare carriers across the country (under the direction of CMS). Errors in reporting modifier 58 occurred most often by general surgeons, ophthalmologists, and orthopaedic surgeons, who were found to be misusing the modifier to bill for postoperative complications treated in the physician office setting. Unless the complications require a return trip to the operating room, these services are included in the global surgical package by Medicare.

the prostate biopsy, a radical perineal prostatectomy with bilateral pelvic lymphadenectomy is performed.

CPT code 55815-58 is submitted.

Example #4:
A partial colon resection (44140) is done, and further treatment (chemotherapy) is needed within the 90-day follow-up period. An implantable venous access port with subQ reservoir (36533) is placed (due to poor peripheral venous circulation) for infusion of chemotherapy.

Submit CPT code 36533-58.

Example #5:
A patient presents for placement of a permanent breast prosthesis. The patient is 30-days postoperative for a mastectomy for breast cancer. The patient is prepped and draped in usual fashion. The subcutaneous tissue expander is removed, and a permanent prosthesis is placed.

Report CPT code 19342-58 for delayed insertion of a breast prosthesis.

Example #6:
A surgeon treated a diabetic (IDDM) patient with advanced circulatory problems. The initial surgery resulted in three gangrenous toes removed from the patient's left foot (28820-T1, 28820-51-T2, 28820-51-T3). During the postoperative period it became necessary to amputate a portion the patient's left foot (28805).

The amputation of the foot was not due to a complication of the first surgery but a more extensive procedure was performed because the wound from the amputation of the toes did not heal due to the underlying disease process. Therefore, the modifier 78 is not appropriate.

Submit 28805-58 modifier. This is an example of using modifier 58 for a more extensive procedure.

59 DISTINCT PROCEDURAL SERVICE

Under certain circumstances, the physician may need to indicate that a procedure or service was distinct or independent from other services performed on the same day. Modifier 59 is used to identify procedures/services that are not normally reported together, but are appropriate under the circumstances. This may represent a different session or patient encounter, different procedure or surgery, different site or organ system, separate incision/excision, separate lesion, or separate injury (or area of injury in extensive injuries) not ordinarily encountered or performed on the same day by the same physician. However, when another already established modifier is appropriate it should be used rather than modifier 59. Only if no more descriptive modifier is available, and the use of modifier 59 best explains the circumstances, should modifier 59 be used.

Using the Modifier Correctly
- Use modifier 59 when billing a combination of codes that would normally not be billed together. This modifier indicates that the ordinarily bundled code represents a service done at a different anatomic site or at a different session on the same date. This may represent:

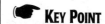

KEY POINT

Use modifier 58 only when the subsequent procedure occurs within the postoperative global surgery period.

KEY POINT

Modifier 59 was established (and replaced the HCPCS Level II temporary modifier GB) to demonstrate that multiple yet distinct services were provided to a patient on the same date of service by the same provider. Because distinct procedures or services rendered on the same day by the same physician cannot be easily identified and therefore properly adjudicated by simply listing the CPT procedure codes, modifier 59 assists the third-party payer or Medicare carrier in applying the appropriate reimbursement protocol. If the modifier is not used in these circumstances, a denial of services may ensue, with the explanation of benefits stating, for instance for Medicare claims, "Medicare does not pay for this service because it is part of another service that was performed at the same time."

—different session or patient encounter

—different procedure or service/same day

—different site or organ system (e.g., a skin graft and an allograft in different locations)

—separate incision/excision

—separate lesion (e.g., a biopsy of skin on the neck is performed at the same session as an excision of a 1.0-cm benign lesion of the face)

—separate injury

- Use modifier 59 only on the procedure designated as the distinct procedural service. The physician needs to document that a procedure or service was distinct or separate from other services performed on the same day.

- Ensure that the medical record documentation is clear as to the separate and distinct procedure before appending modifier 59 to a code. This modifier allows the code to bypass edits; therefore, appropriate documentation must be present in the record. **Note:** Medicare uses the Correct Coding Initiative (CCI) screens when editing claims for possible unbundling. Under CCI screens, specific codes have been identified that should not be billed together.

- When a recurrent hernia requires repair (herniorrhaphy, hernioplasty), bill the appropriate recurrent hernia repair code. A code for incisional hernia repair is not to be billed in addition to the recurrent hernia repair unless a medically necessary incisional hernia repair is performed at a different site. In this case, attach the 59 modifier to the incisional hernia repair code.

- For placement of a tesio catheter, submit CPT code 36533, insertion of implantable venous access device, with or without subcutaneous reservoir, plus code 36491-59, cutdown, over age 2, to allow for the extra procedure and work involved with placement of this type of catheter. Check with your local carrier's medical policy as coverage may vary.

- Modifier 59 is used only if another modifier does not describe the situation more accurately.

Incorrect Use of the Modifier

- Appending modifier 59 to E/M codes.
- Using the modifier 59 as a replacement for modifiers 24, 25, 78, or 79.
- Using modifier 59 when another modifier best describes the distinct service.
- Reporting modifier 59 with modifier 51 on the same CPT code.

Coding Tips

- Modifier 59 is used to indicate that a procedure or service was distinct or independent from other services performed on the same day.
- If there is not a more descriptive modifier available, and the use of modifier 59 best explains the circumstance, then report the service with modifier 59.
- When a procedure or service that is designated as a separate procedure is carried out independently or considered to be unrelated or distinct from the other services provided at the same session, it may be reported by appending the 59 modifier to the specific separate procedure code. This indicates that the procedure is not considered to be a component of another procedure, but instead is a distinct, independent procedure.
- CPT codes for use with modifier 59 unless limited by the payer are 00100–01999, 10021–69990, 70010–79999, 80048–89399, and 90281–99600, when appropriate.

KEY POINT

Use modifier 59 only when the subsequent procedure occurs on the same date as another procedure by the same provider.

Clinical Examples

Example #1:
An arch aortogram and bilateral selective common carotid angiograms are performed by femoral approach. Radiological supervision and interpretation codes are 75650-26 and 75630-26. Results came back with 70 percent stenosis of the right carotid and 95 percent stenosis of the left carotid.

The injection codes are: 36216 and 36215-59. The 59 modifier is used to indicate a different arterial family.

Example #2:
A patient presents for a diagnostic endoscopy that results in a decision to perform an open surgical procedure. The diagnostic endoscopy would be reported using modifier 59 to indicate a distinct diagnostic service when performed at a separate session.

Example #3:
A patient presents with a possible aspiration of a foreign body (food) and a diagnostic bronchoscopy is performed indicating a lobar foreign body. A decision is made to remove the foreign body by thoracotomy.

The same-day open thoracotomy is reported as well as the diagnostic bronchoscopy, which should be appended with the 59 modifier.

Example #4:
A patient presented for the removal of 13 skin tags from his back. At the same session, the physician noted two small lesions (not skin tags) on the patients neck area. Biopsies were taken of each lesion, as each appeared different in its morphology.

CPT codes 11200, 11100-59, and 11101 are submitted. It may also be advisable to append the 59 modifier onto the add on code 11101 in order to show the payer the additional biopsy is not a part of the other procedures.

Example #5:
A scar revision is performed on a painful keloid of a patient's foot, originally caused by stepping on glass five years previously. The original wound was never sutured. The procedure is complex, as the scar measures 3.3 cm and the repair is tedious. During the same session, the physician noted a lesion on the patient's right calf and obtained a skin biopsy.

CPT codes 13132 and 11100-59 are submitted.

62   Two Surgeons

When two surgeons work together as primary surgeons performing distinct part(s) of a procedure, each surgeon should report his/her distinct operative work by adding modifier 62 to the procedure code and any associated add-on code(s) for that procedure as long as both surgeons continue to work together as primary surgeons. Each surgeon should report the cosurgery once using the same procedure code. If additional procedure(s) (including add-on procedure[s]) are performed during the same surgical session, separate code(s) may also be reported with modifier 62.
Note: If a cosurgeon acts as an assistant in the performance of additional procedure(s) during the same surgical session, those services may be reported using separate procedure code(s) with modifier 80 or modifier 82 added, as appropriate

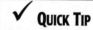

QUICK TIP

There are many possible cosurgery scenarios that are not considered **assistant-at-surgery** situations. CMS instructed all Medicare carriers to adjudicate cosurgeon claims accordingly:

- If two surgeons (each in a different specialty) are required to perform a specific procedure, each surgeon [should] bill for the procedure with a modifier 62. Documentation of the medical necessity for [the services of] two surgeons is required for certain services identified in the MFSDB.
- If a team of surgeons (more than two surgeons of different specialties) is required to perform a specific procedure, each surgeon bills for the procedure [using the] modifier 66. Field 25 of the MFSDB identifies certain [acceptable] services submitted with a 66 modifier which must be sufficiently documented to establish that a [surgical] team was medically necessary. All claims for team surgeons must contain sufficient information to allow pricing **by report**. If surgeons of different specialties are each performing a different procedure (with [different] CPT codes), neither cosurgery nor multiple surgery rules apply (even if the procedures are performed through the same incision). If one of the surgeons performs multiple procedures, the multiple procedure rules apply to that surgeon's services.

Using the Modifier Correctly

- The 62 modifier is added to the procedure number used by each surgeon for reporting services if the services of two physicians are required to manage a specific surgical procedure.

- Modifier 62 is used when the individual skills of physicians with different specialties are required to perform surgery on the patient during the same operative session because of the complex nature of the procedure(s) and/or the patient's condition. In these cases, the physicians are not acting as surgeon and assistant-at-surgery, but rather as cosurgeons (e.g., two surgeons each performing a part of the procedure).

- Submit documentation with claims using modifier 62. Claims for these procedures must include an operative report that supports the need for cosurgeons. If the surgical procedures performed by each physician can be clearly identified, and each surgeon's role is explicitly described within the operative report, then only one operative report is necessary. Otherwise, an operative report dictated by each surgeon is required. If the documentation supports the need for cosurgeons, payment for each physician will be based on the lower of the billed amount or 62.5 percent of the fee schedule amount for Medicare claims.

- Most third-party payers will deny claims by two physicians for cosurgery if the physicians are of the same specialty. On rare occasions Medicare will allow cosurgery claims for physicians with the same specialty designation. In this case, submit claims with the 62 modifier and the 22 modifier for unusual procedural services. Submit the operative report and a cover letter indicating the complex nature of the procedures.

- Although a procedure code may be on the list of procedures for which cosurgery may be covered, the 62 modifier does not apply when two surgeons, regardless of their specialties, perform distinct procedures (different procedure codes). When modifier 62 for cosurgeons is deemed appropriate, payment for an assistant surgeon is usually not allowed (the same is true for team surgeons, modifier 66). However, if it is determined that it was medically necessary to have two surgeons and an assistant surgeon, payment for an assistant surgeon may be allowed.

- Medicare has three classifications for cosurgery:
  - Surgeries that may be paid as cosurgery, but which require documentation to support the medical necessity for the two surgeons. These procedures are reported in the MPFSDB with a "1" in the cosurgery field.
  - Surgeries that may be paid as cosurgery, but do not require documentation, if the two-specialty requirement is met. These procedures are identified in the MPFSDB with a "2" in the cosurgery field.
  - Procedures which may not be billed as cosurgery. These procedures are listed in the MPFSDB with cosurgery indicators of "0" or "9."

Incorrect Use of the Modifier

- Using modifier 62 where the physicians are of the same specialty. Third-party payers typically expect the two surgeons to have different skills. However, there may be instances of medical necessity for two physicians of the same specialty to coperform a procedure. These circumstances require documentation of medical necessity when filing the claims.

- Using modifier 62 when surgeons of different specialties are each performing a different procedure (i.e., reporting different CPT codes even if the procedures are performed through the same incision).

✓ **QUICK TIP**

If a planned procedure requiring cosurgeons is considered not medically necessary under Medicare guidelines, or if there is reason to suspect the cosurgery will be denied due to lack of medical necessity, the Medicare beneficiary must be apprised of this possibility and sign an advance beneficiary notice (ABN), otherwise known as a waiver of liability. This ensures that the patient is aware of his/her financial responsibility. A cosurgery performed and subsequently denied by Medicare for medical necessity reasons cannot be charged to the patient without having, in advance of the procedure(s), a signed ABN on file. (See modifier GA for more information.)

- Using modifier 62 to describe the services of an assistant-at-surgery. See modifiers 80, 81, or 82.

Coding Tips

- Cosurgery refers to a single procedure (same CPT code and add-on codes) requiring two surgeons of different specialties, usually of different skills. When medical necessity exists for both surgeons, Medicare's fee schedule payment amount for the surgery is increased by 25 percent and split equally between the two surgeons.
- It is not always cosurgery when two physicians perform surgery on the same patient during the same operative session. Cosurgery has been performed if the procedures performed are part of, and would be billed under, the same surgical procedure code (e.g., the excision of a pituitary tumor by an otolaryngologist (61548-62) and a neurosurgeon (61548-62).
- Documentation of medical necessity for the two surgeons performing the surgery is required for certain services.
- Surgical procedures in which modifier 62 applies must be billed by each physician with the same date of service and the same procedure code including add-on codes.
- Code ranges for use with modifier 62 (unless limited by the payer) are 10021–69990.

Clinical Examples

Example #1:
When insertion of a pacemaker is performed by a general surgeon and a cardiologist, both physicians should use the appropriate code (33206, 33207, or 33208) with the addition of modifier 62 to indicate that cosurgery was performed. As long as the two-specialty requirements for cosurgery is met, the surgeons should be eligible for reimbursement.

Example #2:
Two surgeons participated in the performance of a laminectomy with removal of abnormal facets and pars interarticularis with decompression of the cauda equina and several nerve roots for lumbar spondylolisthesis.

Submit CPT code 63012-62.

Example #3:
A patient presented for strabismus surgery (two or more vertical muscles for esotropia). This patient has a history of previous eye surgery that did not involve the extraocular muscles. A cosurgeon participated in this procedure due to the procedure's complexity.

Submit CPT code 67316-62 and 67331-62. Use of the -62 modifier in this case requires documentation of medical necessity be sent with the initial claim.

Example #4:
A patient's surgery (for closed fracture of T-1 to T-3) includes arthrodesis of two interspaces of the thoracic spine by anterior interbody technique.

Physician A performs a thoracotomy at the start of the surgical session, and physician B performs the arthrodesis. Upon completion of the arthrodesis, Physician A closes the operative site. Physician A and physician B would report the same CPT code(s)

Hospital ASC and Outpatient Coders
Modifier 62 is not applicable in hospital ASC or hospital outpatient facilities in accordance with CPT's modifiers approved for ambulatory surgery center (ASC) outpatient hospital use.

with the modifier 62 appended, in this instance 22556-62 and 22585-62. Each physician should submit a separate copy of the operative note that explains his or her involvement in the surgery.

63   PROCEDURE PERFORMED ON INFANTS LESS THAN 4KG

Procedures performed on neonates and infants up to a present body weight of 4 kg may involve significantly increased complexity and physician work commonly associated with these patients. This circumstance may be reported by adding the modifier 63 to the procedure number.

Because of the complexity of performing procedures on small infants, a new modifier was added for 2003 to capture services performed on neonates and infants within certain weight limitations.

Using the Modifier Correctly

- Modifier 63 is used when a procedure is performed on an infant or neonate weighing less than 4 kg (8.818 lbs).
- Assign modifier 63 to codes in the surgery section, specifically per the modifier description, procedure codes 20000–69990 only.
- Do not assign modifier 63 to codes where parenthetical notes exclude the use of modifier 63.

Incorrect Use of the Modifier

- Use of the modifier on an infant or neonate over 4 kg.
- Assigning modifier 63 to codes from the evaluation and management, anesthesia, radiology, pathology/laboratory, or medicine sections of the CPT code book.
- Reporting the modifier with codes where instructions indicate modifier 63 is not to be used (e.g., 49491–49496).
- Reporting modifier 63 on procedures performed on a fetus (within the uterine) (e.g., 36430)

Coding Tips

- Add modifier 63 to the basic surgical procedure code when performed on neonates or infants with a weight of 4 kg or less at the time of the procedure.
- Modifier 63 may not be appropriate with certain codes where the description indicates age or weight (e.g., 36510 and 36450).
- Watch for parenthetical notes following certain codes which indicate modifier 63 is not appropriate (e.g., code 36415).
- Follow individual payer guidelines with respect to use of modifier 63.

Clinical Example

Example #1:
A physician performs a push transfusion of blood for an infant age 2 weeks, weighing 3.3 kg.

Submit CPT code 36440-63 (push transfusion, blood, 2 years or under). The addition of modifier 63 tells the third-party payer the physician performed the procedure on an infant less than 4 kg.

Example #2:

A six-week-old infant weighing 3.7 kg with fused anterior sutures of the fontanel presents for repair. The surgeon makes a coronal incision of scalp in a "z" pattern extended. The skin is deflected from the scalp. The fused bilateral sutures are identified and separated. The skin is reapproximated and closed in layered sutures.

Submit code 61552-63 (Craniotomy for craniosynostosis, multiple cranial sutures). The modifier 63 identifies that the infant still weighs less than 4 kg.

66   SURGICAL TEAM

Under some circumstances, highly complex procedures (requiring the concomitant services of several physicians, often of different specialties, plus other highly skilled, specially trained personnel, various types of complex equipment) are carried out under the surgical team concept. Such circumstances may be identified by each participating physician with the addition of the modifier 66 to the basic procedure number used for reporting purposes.

Using the Modifier Correctly

- Modifier 66 is used by each participating surgeon to report his/her services.
- If a highly complex procedure requires the concomitant services of several physicians, often of different specialties, each surgeon would report the same CPT code and modifier 66. For example, CPT code 33945, heart transplant, with or without recipient cardiectomy, represents one major service that combines the work of several physicians and other specially trained personnel. Generally, each physician on a heart transplant team performs the same portion of the transplant surgery each time it is performed. Each physician would report code 33945-66.
- If the surgery is billed with a modifier 66 and the documentation supports the need for team surgeons, claims will be considered by report. All claims for team surgery must contain sufficient information to support the medical necessity for a surgical team. Hard copies of this documentation should be sent with claims.

Incorrect Use of the Modifier

- Using modifier 66 when other specially trained personnel are not involved.

Coding Tips

- The modifier 66 is added to the basic procedure when the concomitant services of several physicians, plus other highly skilled, specially trained personnel and various types of complex equipment are required to perform a procedure.
- CPT codes for use with the modifier 66 unless limited by the payer are 10021–69990, when appropriate.

Clinical Examples

Example #1:

A surgical team of three surgeons were required to perform a vertebral corpectomy, complete, with a combined thoracolumbar approach with decompression of the spinal cord, cauda equina and nerve roots of the lower thoracic spine for HNP of the thoracic vertebrae. This surgery involved two segments.

©2003 Ingenix, Inc.
CPT only ©2003 American Medical Association. All Rights Reserved.

Documentation will be required by each billing surgeon for this procedure and the medical necessity for three surgeons acting as a surgical team and not cosurgeons or assistant-at-surgery must be clearly documented.

Each surgeon should submit claims with CPT codes 63087-66 and 63088-66. CPT code 63088 is not also appended with modifier 51, multiple procedures, because it is an add-on code.

Example #2:
An operation was scheduled for extracorporeal bench surgery for renal artery thrombosis. A nephrolithotomy was also performed. This procedure will require a team of surgeons to successfully complete. Each surgeon should submit CPT codes 50380-66 and 50060-66-51 to denote a team approach.

76   REPEAT PROCEDURE BY SAME PHYSICIAN

The physician may need to indicate that a procedure or service was repeated subsequent to the original procedure or service. This circumstance may be reported by adding modifier 76 to the repeated procedure/service.

Using the Modifier Correctly

- Modifier 76 is appended to a code when the same physician repeats the same service, sometimes on the same day. This modifier can be used whenever the circumstances warrant this information.
- Use this modifier to indicate that a repeat procedure was necessary and that it does not represent a duplicate bill for the original surgery or service.

Incorrect use of the modifier

- Using modifier 76 to indicate repositioning or replacement 14 days after the initial insertion or replacement of an existing pacemaker or defibrillator. Modifier 76 is not reported with pacemaker or defibrillator codes after 14 days, as these are considered new, not repeat services.
- As an example, procedure codes such as 17000, 17003, and 17004 by description indicate multiple procedures on the same day, and therefore, use of modifier 76 would be inappropriate.

Coding Tips

- The modifier 76 is added to the repeat service to indicate that a procedure or service was repeated subsequent to the original service. An explanation of the medical necessity for the repeat procedure is necessary (e.g., repeat x-ray performed after thoracotomy tube placement).
- For repeated clinical laboratory tests on the same day, see modifier 91 in the pathology and laboratory chapter.
- CPT codes for use with modifier 76, unless limited by the payer, are 10021–69990, 70010–79999, and 90281–99600, when appropriate.

Clinical Examples

Example #1
Lacrimal punctum plugs are used to close the puncta located at the inner corners of the eyes. Procedure code 68761 identifies the closure of a single punctum. If the procedure is performed on both eyes, report 68761-50. In situations where two puncta are treated in the same eye, submit code 68761-76-RT or -LT eye. In

QUICK TIP

Hospital ASC and Outpatient Coders
Medicare's instructions for Modifiers 76 and 77 in hospital ASC or hospital outpatient facilities include in the definition procedures "repeated in a separate operative session on the same calendar day." Use modifier 76 for same physician/same day and modifier 77 for another physician/same day. The procedure must be the same procedure.

situations where two puncta are treated in both eyes, submit code 68761-RT or -LT on the first line and 68761-RT or -LT-76 on the second line. If four puncta are closed, the physician should bill 68761-50 on the first line and 68761-76-50 on the next line.

Example #2:

A 68-year-old female was in an assisted living center when fire erupted. She sustained severe inhalation burns. The patient is found to have extreme difficulty breathing and a suction bronchoscopy is performed. Due to the severity of her condition, the next day a suction bronchoscopy is performed at 7:30 a.m., and repeated at 5:30 p.m. by the same physician.

Report 31645 for the initial bronchoscopy. For the second day report 31646 for the first procedure and 31646-76 for the second bronchoscopy.

77   REPEAT PROCEDURE BY ANOTHER PHYSICIAN

The physician may need to indicate that a basic procedure or service performed by another physician had to be repeated. This situation may be reported by adding modifier 77 to the repeated procedure/service.

Using the Modifier Correctly
- Modifier 77 is appended to a CPT code when the same service (same CPT code), which was already performed by another physician, is repeated by another physician. Sometimes this occurs on the same date of service. This modifier can be used whenever the circumstances warrant this information.

Incorrect Use of the Modifier
- Using modifier 77 to indicate repositioning or replacement 14 days after the initial insertion or replacement of an existing pacemaker or defibrillator. Modifier 77 is not reported with pacemaker or defibrillator codes after 14 days because these are considered new, not repeat services.

Coding Tips
- Modifier 77 is added to the repeated service to indicate that a basic procedure performed by another physician needed to be repeated by a different physician. An explanation of the medical necessity for the repeat service is necessary.
- Modifier 77 is used to show the third-party payer that the procedure or service was actually rendered again. This will help them to distinguish claim submissions from those which are inadvertently duplicated billings.
- Modifier 77 does not guarantee reimbursement of repeated services, as individual third-party payer regulations (such as medical necessity) are still applicable.
- CPT codes for use with modifier 77, unless limited by the payer, are 10021–69990, 70010–79999, and 90281–99600, when appropriate.

Clinical Example
A patient was prepped and draped for a thoracocentesis of the left lower chest. The presenting diagnosis was carcinoma of the left breast with bone and pulmonary metastases, as well as pleural effusion in the left pleural cavity.

A #18 needle connected to a three-stop cock and a 30 cc syringe was then inserted into the pleural space and aspirate of approximately 1400 cc of cloudy brownish fluid consistent with a malignant pleural effusion was obtained. The fluid was sent for cytology.

©2003 Ingenix, Inc.
CPT only ©2003 American Medical Association. All Rights Reserved.

The following day, the patient underwent repeat thoracentesis by another physician.

CPT code 32000-77 is submitted.

78 RETURN TO OPERATING ROOM FOR A RELATED PROCEDURE DURING THE POSTOPERATIVE PERIOD

The physician may need to indicate that another procedure was performed during the postoperative period of the initial procedure. When this subsequent procedure is related to the first, and requires the use of the operating room, it may be reported by adding the modifier 78 to the related procedure. (For repeat procedures on the same day, see 76.)

Using the Modifier Correctly

- Using modifier 78 when treatment for complications requires a return trip to the operating room. Use the CPT code that best describes the procedure performed during the return trip.
- Modifier 78 is used on surgical codes only to indicate that another procedure was performed during the postoperative period of the initial procedure, was related to the first and required the use of the operating room.
- If the patient is returned to the operating room after the initial operative session, even if on the same day as the original surgery, for one or more additional procedures as a result of complications from the original surgery, use the 78 modifier.

Incorrect Use of the Modifier

- Using modifier 78 on the procedure code when the original surgery is repeated. If the identical procedure was repeated by the same physician use modifier 76.
- Only using modifier 78 for complications of surgery. The CPT definition for this modifier does not limit its use to treatment for complications.
- Using this modifier to bill Medicare for a procedure not performed in the OR (unless the patient's condition was so critical there would be insufficient time for transportation to an operating room).

Coding Tips

- Modifier 78 is added to the procedure code when the subsequent procedure is related to the first and requires the use of an operating room. Failure to use this modifier when appropriate may result in denial of the subsequent surgery.
- If a CPT code exists for the related procedure, append 78 to it. If no CPT code exists for the related procedure, append the modifier to an unlisted procedure code. For Medicare patients, payment is limited to the amount allotted for intraoperative services only. [Note: For each surgical CPT code, most third-party payers have established a certain reimbursement percentage for each of the three components (i.e., preoperative, intraoperative and postoperative).]
- Do not use modifier 78 if treatment for postoperative complications did not require a return trip to the operating room.
- A new postoperative period does not begin with the use of the 78 modifier.
- An operating room is defined by CMS as a place of service specifically equipped and staffed for the sole purpose of performing procedures. This includes cardiac catheterization suites, laser suites and endoscopy suites. It does not include a patient's room, a minor treatment room, a recovery room or an intensive care unit.

✓ QUICK TIP

Modifier 78, among others, was the recent target of an investigation by various Medicare carriers across the country (under the direction of CMS). Errors in reporting modifier 78 occurred most often by ophthalmologists, who were found to be misusing the modifier to bill for postoperative complications treated in the physician office setting. Unless the complications require a return trip to the operating room, these services are included in the global surgical package by Medicare.

- CPT codes for use with the modifier 78 are 10021–69990 and 90281–99600, when appropriate.

Clinical Examples

Example #1:
A single vessel coronary graft 33510 is performed. In the patient's room that evening it is noted his vital signs are unstable, and it is observed that hemorrhagic complications following the surgery have occurred. The patient is returned to the operating room on the same date to locate and control the source of hemorrhage.

Submit CPT codes 33510 and 35820-78.

Example #2:
A femoral-popliteal nonautogenous bypass graft (35656) is placed. Infection is noted in the lower extremity within the follow-up period (during the 90 days after the surgery) of the bypass graft. The patient is returned to the operating room for exploration.

CPT code 35860-78 is submitted for the subsequent exploration procedure.

Example #3:
A patient presents for hernia repair with ligation of spermatic veins for varicocele. An incision is made in the affected area and the spermatic cords are exposed. The cord is brought up into the incision and the structures of the cord are dissected, the veins identified and ligated. The hernia is repaired and the dilated veins are ligated through a separate incision in the scrotum. The patient is sent to the recovery room in satisfactory condition. Later in the day, the patient's operative site bleeds and requires a return to the operating room to stop the bleeding.

Submit CPT code 35840-78, for the exploration for postoperative hemorrhage, thrombosis or infection, abdomen.

Example #4
OPERATIVE REPORT:

Preoperative Diagnosis: Abdominal aortic aneurysm

Postoperative Diagnosis: Same

Operation Performed: Resection of abdominal aortic aneurysm, placement of a bifurcated Hemashield graft, 18 x 9 mm, both iliac arteries.

Anesthesia: General endotracheal

Indications: The patient is a 79-year-old gentleman who was seen by me last fall for an abdominal aortic aneurysm. It had reached a dimension of 5.8 cm by ultrasound. I recommended surgery for the patient but he declined at that time. His wife became concerned and encouraged him to see me again. He is admitted at this time for resection of the aneurysm. A CT scan confirmed the ultrasound findings.

The risks and benefits of the operation were carefully explained to the patient including bleeding, infection, death, stroke, cardiac difficulties, myocardial infarction, arrhythmias, impotence, etc. The patient and his wife had all their

Hospital ASC and Outpatient Coders
Medicare's instructions for modifiers 78 and 79 in hospital ASC or hospital outpatient facilities include in the definition procedures "return to the operating room on the same day." Use modifier 78 for a procedure related to the initial procedure on the same day and modifier 79 for a procedure on the same day that is unrelated to the initial procedure.

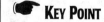

Categories 996–999 in ICD-9-CM, "Complications of Surgical Care, Not Elsewhere Classified," identify many postoperative complications.

questions answered. The patient was taken to the operating room for resection of the abdominal aortic aneurysm.

Procedure: After obtaining adequate general endotracheal anesthesia, the patient was prepped and draped in the usual sterile fashion.

A standard midline incision was created and the abdomen was explored. Adhesions were taken down from his previous operation. His retroperitoneum was opened. All of his colon and retroperitoneal structures appeared normal. The aneurysm was found to be saccular in nature in the midportion of the abdominal aorta. The proximal aorta was calcified up to the renal arteries. The iliacs were soft on the right and calcified on the left down to the bifurcation, at which point the iliacs again became very soft.

Heparin was administered and allowed to circulate. After an adequate circulation time, the iliac arteries were clamped first followed by the neck of the aneurysm below the renal arteries. This was actually not the neck of the aneurysm but the proximal extent of the calcium. The aneurysm was then opened. The aneurysm was opened up proximally and then down onto both iliac arteries. The contents were extracted.

Both iliac arteries were allowed to back bleed. We actually obtained debris out of the left iliac artery. We, therefore, repeated this procedure several times during the operation. An 18 x 9 mm Hemashield graft was chosen. The proximal portion of the aorta was prepared and the anastomosis created in standard fashion with running 3-0 prolene suture. We paid careful attention to the technical aspects of the operation because of the calcium and the poor quality of the proximal anatomic aorta.

The clamp was released and the graft filled. Two repair sutures were required anteriorly at the suture line. After these were placed, the suture line was completely hemostatic. The graft was allowed to bleed freely into the abdomen for a couple of beats to clear the graft of any debris.

The graft was then cut to length on both sides and both iliac arteries fashioned to receive an anastomosis. As mentioned, the left iliac was prepared beyond the calcium. The left iliac anastomosis was then performed with running 3-0 prolene suture. This went well. This was de-aired and allowed to bleed freely to free up any debris. It was then tied down and secured. The left leg was opened without any hemodynamic instability.

The right graft was then created in an end-to-side fashion. The anastomosis went very well. The iliac was back-bled and allowed to de-air, and we also irrigated the anastomotic area. After this was performed, the anastomosis was tied down completely and flow established into the right leg as well. A repair stitch was required on the left iliac anastomosis, but other than that, flow was established without difficulty. The femoral pulses were strong bilaterally.

The area was copiously irrigated with antibiotic solution. Heparin was reversed by a 50 percent dose. After hemostasis was achieved, the aneurysm was closed over the anterior wall of the graft. This was only possible in the midportion where the aorta was actually aneurysmal. The retroperitoneum was then closed over the graft itself. The proximal suture line was covered completely with peritoneum.

The abdominal contents were placed in correct anatomic position. The abdomen was irrigated with antibiotic solution. Closure was routine with a heavy prolene running suture. The subcutaneous tissue was closed with 2-0 vicryl and the skin with 3-0 vicryl. Each layer of closure was copiously irrigated with antibiotic solution.

At the end of the procedure, the final instrument counts were correct times two. The patient tolerated the procedure well. Pulses were easily palpable in both feet. The patient was transferred to the thoracic intensive care unit in stable and satisfactory condition.

CPT code 35102 is submitted.

The patient was three days postoperative when he suddenly complained of severe abdominal pain. Inspection of the surgical wound revealed rupture of the suture lines and total loss of incision approximation. The patient was returned to the OR for closure of a wound dehiscence.

CPT code 13160-78 is submitted.

79   Unrelated Procedure or Service by the Same Physician During the Postoperative Period

The physician may need to indicate that the performance of a procedure or service during the postoperative period was unrelated to the original procedure. This circumstance may be reported by using the modifier 79. (For repeat procedures on the same day, see modifier 76.)

Using the Modifier Correctly
- Modifier 79 is used on surgical codes only to indicate that an unrelated procedure was performed by the same physician during the postoperative period of the original procedure.

Incorrect Use of the Modifier
- Using the modifier 79 to describe a related procedure performed in a postoperative period, by the same surgeon.

Coding Tips
- Modifier 79 is used to indicate that the procedure performed by the physician is unrelated to the original service or procedure, a different diagnosis code should be reported. Failure to use this modifier when appropriate may result in denial of the subsequent surgery.
- It is important that each line item include the necessary modifier when appropriate. For example, if the physician has performed two unrelated surgical procedures that fall in the postoperative period of another surgery the physician performed, apply the modifier 79 to both surgery codes, not just the first.
- CPT codes for use with the modifier 79 (unless limited by the payer) are 10021–69990, 70010–79999, and 90281–99600, when appropriate.

Clinical Examples

Example #1:
A total knee replacement (27447) is done. Within the 90-day follow-up period for the knee replacement, care for a Colles' fracture of the wrist (25620) is provided.

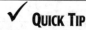

Hospital ASC and Outpatient Coders
Medicare's instructions for Modifiers 78 and 79 in hospital ASC or hospital outpatient facilities include in the definition procedures "return to the operating room on the same day." Use modifier 78 for a procedure related to the initial procedure on the same day and modifier 79 for a procedure on the same day that is unrelated to the initial procedure.

The federal Medicare program includes specific medical and/or surgical care for postoperative complications as included within the standard global surgical package (i.e., for which there is no additional payment). Patient care included in the global surgical package is defined as "additional medical and surgical services required of the surgeon during the postoperative period of the surgery because of complications which do not require additional trips to the operating room."

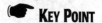

When billing for an unrelated procedure by the same physician during the postoperative period of an original procedure, a new postoperative period will begin with the subsequent procedure.

Modifier 79 with code 25620 is submitted.

Example #2:
A patient, having had a femoral-popliteal graft performed one week previously, presents to the same physician with symptoms of acute renal failure. He is admitted for care but does not respond to the prescribed treatment. His physician discusses the possibility of hemodialysis with the patient and his family. They agree that it is a viable option. The physician inserts a cannula for hemodialysis.

Submit CPT code 36810-79, since the insertion of the cannula for hemodialysis was not related to the femoral-popliteal graft that was performed earlier.

Example #3:
A patient is 60 days postoperative for an excision of a tumor of the upper left arm (CPT code 24077). He presents to the same general surgeon complaining of a persistent pain across his abdomen. The pain has increased in severity and the patient is now complaining of nausea. After an examination the patient undergoes emergency surgery for a ruptured appendix.

CPT code 44960-79 is submitted.

80 ASSISTANT SURGEON

Surgical assistant services may be identified by adding the modifier 80 to the usual procedure number(s).

Using the Modifier Correctly
- Use modifier 80 on the appropriate procedure code(s). The code or codes must match that reported by the primary surgeon.
- If an assistant-at-surgery is used in a procedure also requiring the skills of two surgeons (modifier 62 or 66), report modifier 80 on the surgical assistant's claim and submit documentation supporting the medical necessity for the use of the surgical assistant.
- Modifier 80 can also be used on claims with other surgical modifiers, such as 50 and 51.

Incorrect Use of the Modifier
- Using modifier 80 with certain surgical procedures that are not covered for a surgical assistant. These procedures are not covered by Medicare Part B for surgical assistance, and providers cannot charge the patient for these services under any circumstances.
- Using modifier 80 when modifier 82 is more appropriate in a teaching setting. (See modifier 82.)

Coding Tips
- The modifier 80 is added to the usual procedure code(s) for surgical assistance services.
- Even though under many circumstances a surgeon may request or require the services of an assistant-at-surgery, Medicare will only pay for services of the assistant if the surgery is medically necessary and the surgery is approved for assistant-at-surgery coverage. Medicare's payment criteria states payment cannot be made to an assistant-at-surgery when an assistant in less is used in than 5 percent of the cases nationally.

✓ **QUICK TIP**

Physicians are prohibited from charging a Medicare beneficiary for assistant-at-surgery services for procedures not covered by this benefit. Physicians who knowingly and willfully violate this rule may be subject to penalties and/or sanctions under the Medicare program and the Social Security Act, as well as fraud and abuse penalties under the Health Insurance Portability and Accountability Act (HIPAA) of 1996 and the Balanced Budget Act (BBA) of 1997.

Chapter 3: Surgery

- To determine if a surgical procedure is subject to the assistant-at-surgery restriction, refer to the Medicare physician fee schedule data base (MPFSDB).
  —an assistant surgery indicator of "0" identifies procedures that are restricted and not payable.
  —an indicator of "1" denotes procedures that would require medical necessity documentation in order for Medicare to pay for an assistant-at-surgery. A waiver should be signed (see modifier GA).
  —an indicator of "2" denotes a procedure that will allow payment for an assistant-at-surgery for this procedure.
- CPT codes for use with the 80 modifier are appropriate codes in the surgery section (10021–69990), unless limited by the third-party payer.

Clinical Examples

Example #1:

A physician takes down and closes an intestinal cutaneous fistula by making an abdominal incision. The bowel is mobilized and the fistula is identified and taken down from the abdominal wall and skin. The segment of bowel containing the fistula is resected and the bowel is reapproximated with staples. The abdominal wall incision is closed and the incision is dressed.

The primary operating surgeon would submit CPT code 44640 and the physician acting as the assistant surgeon would report 44640-80.

Example #2:

Surgeon: Dr. Wurthers

Assistant Surgeon: Dr. Black

Preoperative Diagnosis: Distal urethral stricture, status post multiple urethroplasties for hypospadias

Postoperative diagnosis: Same

Operation performed: First stage Johannsen's urethroplasty, cystourethroscopy

Indications: This is a 35-year-old male with a history of congenital hypospadias defect. The patient has undergone several urethroplasties but has developed recurrent stenosis of the distal urethra with significant scarring from the previous procedures. Dr. Black will assist with the surgical procedure(s).

Procedure: The patient was prepped and draped in the dorsal lithotomy position. The meatus was probed with a bougie-a-boule sounds. The meatus was found to be recessed and displaced to the patient's left side and was very stenotic, only accepting the 8-French sound. The strictured area was dilated to 14-French but could not be dilated further due to the marked stricture.

The distal urethra was then incised by cutting over a VanBuren sound through the penile skin and bulbospongiosus tissue until the lumen was reached. The incision was extended until healthy urethra was reached, which was roughly a length of approximately 2 cm.

©2003 Ingenix, Inc.
CPT only ©2003 American Medical Association. All Rights Reserved.

The urethroplasty was then completed by removing the redundant skin on the patient's right side to move the meatus into a more medial position. The meatus then readily calibrated to 24-French following the urethroplasty.

A cystourethroscope was introduced revealing a normal prostatic urethra. The bladder also appeared unremarkable. An antibiotic ointment was placed over the urethroplasty, and several cc of a 0.25 percent Marcaine solution were injected subcutaneously around the penile shaft for anesthetic purposes. The patient was then transferred to the recovery room in good condition.

CPT code 53400-80 for the assistant-at-surgery is submitted.

81 Minimum Assistant Surgeon

Minimum surgical assistant services are identified by adding the modifier 81 to the usual procedure number.

Using the Modifier Correctly
- Modifier 81 is used when the services of a second or third assistant surgeon are required during a procedure. Payers have varied interpretations on how or if modifier 81 should be used. Many do not recognize this modifier.
- Use modifier 81 when the assistant-at-surgery is not present for the entire procedure.

Incorrect Use of the Modifier
- Using modifier 81 to describe a full assist. See modifiers 80 and 82.

Coding Tips
- At times, while a primary operating physician may plan to perform a surgical procedure alone, during an operation circumstances may arise that require the services of an assistant surgeon for a relatively short time. Append modifier 81 to the surgical procedure when the second surgeon provides minimal assistance.
- Modifier 81 does not appear on the MPFSDB. It is rarely recognized by CMS (except in extreme cases). Check with your other third-party carriers to determine reporting and reimbursement policies for this modifier.
- CPT codes for use with modifier 81 are appropriate codes in the surgery section (10021–69990), unless limited by the third-party payer.

82 Assistant Surgeon (When a Qualified Resident Is Not Available)

The unavailability of a qualified resident surgeon is a prerequisite for use of modifier 82 appended to the usual procedure code number(s).

Using the Modifier Correctly
- Modifier 82 is used to indicate a surgical assist when a qualified resident is not available. Many hospitals have residency programs and Medicare Part B will not make payment when a resident is used as an assistant. Medicare Part B only allows use of the 82 modifier for services rendered by a medical doctor. The location where the services were rendered must be shown in item 32 of the CMS-1500 claim form.

Quick Tip

Modifier 81 is not intended, nor is it to be used, to bill nonphysician assistants at surgery who do not meet criteria for payment as a provider under Medicare Part B. Medicare Part B does not recognize for payment scrub technicians, certified surgical assistants, registered nurses, medical assistants, etc., as assistants-at-surgery. The payment for nonphysician assistants who do not qualify to bill Medicare Part B is considered included (bundled) in the payment to the hospital or ASC, and should not be unbundled and billed either to a carrier or to a beneficiary.

Quick Tip

The Medicare fee schedule amount for an assistant-at-surgery is 16 percent of the amount allowed for a nonassisted procedure. Medicare payment for assistant-at-surgery does not include preoperative or postoperative visits by the assistant surgeon. For nonparticipating assistant surgeons, the billed amount cannot exceed the limiting charge (15 percent more than the MPFSDB amount) reduced to 16 percent.

- Payment may be made for the services of an assistant-at-surgery, regardless of the availability of a qualified resident, when one of the following conditions exists:

  —exceptional medical circumstances (i.e., emergency life-threatening situations such as multiple traumatic injuries requiring immediate treatment)

  —the primary surgeon has an across-the-board policy of never involving residents in the preoperative, operative or postoperative care of his or her patients (This often occurs when community physicians have no involvement in a hospital's graduate medical education program.)

  —complex medical procedures, including multistage transplant surgery, which may require a team of physicians

- When payment may be made for the services of assistants-at-surgery, regardless of the availability of a qualified resident, use modifier 80, 62, or 66 as appropriate (Use the same procedure code as the surgeon with modifier 82.

- When using modifier 82, the assistant must provide documentation (certification) stating that a qualified resident was not available for this procedure and why the resident was not available (The documentation can be submitted in the electronic claim free-form text area, by attachment, or in the body of the paper claim form [item 19].)

Incorrect Use of the Modifier
- Using modifier 82 modifier on a consistent basis by physicians in teaching facilities. This practice would raise a flag indicating potential abuse.
- Using modifier 82 when a qualified resident is available.

Coding Tips
- The unavailability of a qualified resident surgeon is a prerequisite for use of modifier 82 appended to the procedure code(s). In a teaching hospital, Medicare presumes that a resident is available unless certification is on file that attests otherwise.
- CMS has strict guidelines regarding the use of this modifier. Certification for its use must be on file for each claim, and some carriers require the certification accompany each claim. The certification statement is as follows: "I understand that section 1842 of the Social Security Act prohibits Medicare Part B payment for the services of an assistant-at-surgery in teaching hospitals when qualified residents are available to furnish such services. I certify that the services for which payment is claimed were medically necessary and that no qualified resident was available to perform the service. I further understand that these services are subject to postpayment review by the Medicare carrier."
- Modifier 82 indicates one of the criteria (see below) exists and that an assistant surgeon should be paid.
- CPT codes for use with the modifier 82, unless limited by the payer, are appropriate codes in the surgery section (10021–69990).

Clinical Example
A neurosurgeon, who is a teaching physician in a teaching facility, has a new patient with multiple brain tumors that are life-threatening. The physician elects to perform surgery in an attempt to save the patient's life. Since the operation is one that requires an assistant-at-surgery and the neurosurgeon realizes that no resident is qualified to assist him with this type of surgery, another neurosurgeon is called in to assist.

©2003 Ingenix, Inc.
CPT only ©2003 American Medical Association. All Rights Reserved.

Since the teaching facility did not have a qualified resident to assist the neurosurgeon, report the 82 modifier on the assistant's claim to ensure payment.

99 MULTIPLE MODIFIERS

Under certain circumstances two or more modifiers may be necessary to completely delineate a service. In such situations modifier 99 should be added to the basic procedure, and the other applicable modifiers may be listed as part of the description of the service.

Using the Modifier Correctly

- If the third-party payer's computer system accepts multiple modifiers on the same line, then modifier 99 is not needed. If the system does not, report the 99 modifier as follows:
  —the modifier 99 is placed after a selected CPT code to illustrate to the payer that multiple modifiers apply to the service(s). Use modifier 99 on the basic service. Enter on the CMS-1500 claim form all applicable additional modifiers in item 19. If modifier 99 is entered on multiple line items, all applicable modifiers for each line item containing a 99 modifier should be listed as follows: 1 = (mod), where the number 1 represents the specific line item and mod represents all modifiers applicable to the referenced line item. For electronic submissions, the additional modifiers should be listed in the extra narrative field, record HAO, field 05.0, positions 40 through 320. If the individual modifiers are not identified, the claim may be denied.

Incorrect Use of the Modifier

- Applying modifier 99 to a code with either one additional or no additional modifiers.

Coding Tips

- Modifier 99 is added to the basic service when more than two modifiers are needed to describe a service. The additional modifiers should be included with the claim (item 19 on paper claim submissions, or the appropriate message in the free-form area on electronic submissions).
- Before using modifier 99, check with your third-party payers regarding their rules for its use.
- CPT codes for use with the modifier 99 unless limited by the payer are 10021–69990, 70010–79999, and 90281–99600, when appropriate.

KEY POINT

Submitting 99 by Electronic Claim

When submitting modifier 99, multiple modifiers, by electronic claims, many third-party payers, including some Medicare carriers, require the modifier 99 in the first modifier field, the second modifier in the second modifier field, and the remaining modifiers in the narrative (HAO) record.

When submitting only two modifiers or less and, therefore, not reporting the modifier 99, continue to use only the first and second modifier fields.

Chapter 4: Radiology

22 UNUSUAL PROCEDURAL SERVICES

When the service(s) provided is greater than that usually required for the listed procedure, it may be identified by adding modifier 22 to the usual procedure number. A report may also be appropriate. **Note:** This modifier is not to be used to report procedure(s) complicated by adhesion formation, scarring, and/or alteration of normal landmarks due to late effects of prior surgery, irradiation, infection, very low weight (i.e., neonates and infants less than 4kg), or trauma.

Using the Modifier Correctly
- Modifier 22 is appended to the basic CPT procedure code when the service(s) provided is greater than usually required for the listed procedure. Use of modifier 22 allows the claim to undergo individual consideration.
- Modifier 22 is used to identify an increment of work that is infrequently encountered with a particular procedure and is not described by another code.
- Modifier 22 is generally not appended to a radiology code. If a rare circumstance does occur, submit detailed documentation with a cover letter from the radiologist or other provider.
- The frequent reporting of modifier 22 has prompted many carriers to simply ignore it.
- Modifier 22 is used with computerized tomography (CT) numbers when additional slices are required or a more detailed examination is necessary. However, this is subject to payer discretion. Many payers will not allow additional reimbursement for additional CT slices.

Incorrect Use of the Modifier
- Appending this modifier to a radiology code without justification in the medical record documenting an unusual occurrence. Because of its overuse, many payers do not acknowledge this modifier.
- Using this modifier on a routine basis; to do so would most certainly cause scrutiny of submitted claims and may result in an audit.
- Using modifier 22 to indicate that the radiology procedure was performed by a specialist; specialty designation does not warrant use of the 22 modifier.
- Using modifier 22 when more x-rays views are taken than actually specified by the CPT code description. This is incorrect, especially when the code descriptor reads "complete" (e.g., 70130, 70321, 73110, etc.). Complete means any number of views taken of the body site.

Coding Tips
- Using modifier 22 identifies the service as one that requires individual consideration and manual review.
- Overuse of modifier 22 could trigger a carrier audit. Carriers monitor the use of this modifier very carefully. The 22 modifier should be used only when sufficient documentation is present in the medical record.
- A Medicare claim submitted with modifier 22 is forwarded to the carrier medical review staff for review and pricing. With sufficient documentation of medical necessity, increased payment may result.

Hospital ASC and Outpatient Coders
Modifier 22 is not applicable in hospital ASC or hospital outpatient facilities in accordance with CPT modifiers approved for ambulatory surgery center (ASC) outpatient hospital use.

Claims submitted to Medicare, Medicaid, and other third-party payers containing modifier 22 for unusual procedural services that do not have attached supporting documentation that illustrates the unusual distinction of the services will generally be processed as if the procedure codes were not appended with this modifier. Some third-party payers might suspend the claims and request additional information from the provider, but this is the exception rather than the rule.

Do not bombard the Medicare carrier or other third-party payer with unnecessary documentation. All attachments to the claim for justification of the unusual services should explain the unusual circumstances in a concise, clear manner. The information for the justification of unusual services should be easy to locate within the attached documentation. Highlight this information, if necessary, to facilitate the medical reviewer's access to the pertinent supporting data.

- For a nonparticipating physician, the limiting charge provisions (see next bullet) apply to services that are billed with modifier 22 and to all claims submitted to Medicare as a secondary payer, if the services billed are those on the physician fee schedule and are subject to charge limits. In all cases the limiting charge cannot exceed a percentage of the allowable amount. This is the case even in instances where the allowance amount will not be known until the claim is individually priced.

- A claim with modifier 22 will be processed on a by-report basis and will cause the claim processing to be delayed. In these cases, Medicare will consider the unusual nature of the service and, if they believe a charge above the fee schedule is justified, will approve an amount that recognizes the additional services. This in effect becomes a higher-than-usual fee schedule amount for the service. The approved amount (or higher fee schedule amount) is the basis of the limiting charge calculation for modifier 22 services. Therefore, if the billed amount exceeds Medicare's approved amount by more than 15 percent, you must make an adjustment or a refund to the patient in order to meet the limiting charge requirements of the law. Because the exact limiting charge on these cases is not known until an allowable amount decision is made, Medicare would not consider these cases as knowing or willful violations, provided the physician made the appropriate adjustments or refunds.

- CPT codes for use with modifier 22 are 00100–01999, 10021–69990, 70010–79999, 80048–89399, and 90281–99600 unless limited by the payer.

Clinical Examples

Example #1:

A brain imaging, complete study with vascular flow, was performed. The patient was very apprehensive and anxious. This procedure was delayed several times due to patient movement and noncompliance with instructions. The patient complained of severe headache. The patient's blood pressure was elevated and responded to medication. The work involved in performing this procedure was double what is normally required. The radiologist documented the procedure in detail.

CPT code 78606-26-22 is submitted with a cover letter to the carrier explaining the rationale for use of 22 modifier in this case.

Example #2:

A 16-year-old female presented for an intravenous pyelography with KUB and tomography. During the procedure, the patient complained of shortness of breath and nausea. There did not appear to be an allergic reaction, so the procedure was cautiously continued. The patient was extremely apprehensive and the procedure was prolonged by 70 minutes beyond its usual duration.

CPT code 74400-22 is sumbitted with detailed documentation and a cover letter with the initial claim.

26   PROFESSIONAL COMPONENT

Certain procedures are a combination of a physician component and a technical component. When the physician component is reported separately, the service may be identified by adding the modifier 26 to the usual procedure number.

Using the Modifier Correctly
- Modifier 26 is appended to the procedure code to report only the professional component.
- Modifier 26 is used in those instances during which a physician provides the interpretation of the diagnostic test/study performed. The interpretation of the diagnostic test/study has to be separate, distinct, identifiable, written, and signed.
- If a diagnostic test or radiology service is billed using separate professional (modifier 26) and technical (modifier TC) components, the sum of the allowances for both components will not exceed the allowance for the global procedure for many third-party payers.

Incorrect Use of the Modifier
- Using modifiers 26 and TC (except for purchased diagnostic tests) when a diagnostic test or radiology service is performed globally (both components are performed by the same provider). When a global service is performed, the code representing the complete service should be reported without modifiers. The payment for the global service will reflect the allowances for both components.
- Using modifier 26 for a reread of results of an interpretation initially provided by another physician.
- Using both modifier 26 indicating that only the professional portion of the service was provided and modifier 52 for reduced service. It is not necessary to use 52 since the professional modifier already indicates that only a portion of the complete service was performed.

Coding Tips
- Certain procedures are a combination of a physician component and a technical component (TC). To report the physician component separately, add modifier 26 to the procedure code.
- In order to use the professional component modifier (26), the provider must prepare a written report that includes findings, relevant clinical issues and, if appropriate, comparative data. This report must be available if requested by the carrier. A review of the diagnostic procedure findings, without a written report similar to that which would be prepared by a specialist in the field, does not meet the conditions for modifier use. The review of the findings, usually documented in the medical record or on a machine-generated report as "fx-tibia" or "EKG-WNL" does not suffice as a separately identifiable report and therefore is not eligible for payment. These types of procedure review notes should be bundled into any E/M code billed for that date. If a postpayment review of the medical record reveals that no separate, written interpretive report exists, overpayment recoveries may be sought.
- CPT codes for use with modifier 26 are 10040–69979, 70010–79999, 80048–89399, and 90281–99600 unless limited by the payer.

Clinical Examples

Example #1:
A patient presented to the emergency department (ED) with complaints of severe left wrist pain after falling onto her outstretched hand. X-rays confirmed an ulnar shaft fracture. The radiologist interpreted the wrist x-ray by written report (73110; complete, minimum of three views). The ED physician performed an examination and following the encounter, the physician performed closed treatment of the ulnar shaft fracture, without manipulation.

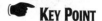

KEY POINT

In order to use a PC modifier 26, the provider must prepare a written report that includes findings, relevant clinical issues, and if appropriate, comparative data.

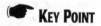

KEY POINT

There are certain procedure codes that describe and represent only the professional component portion of a procedure or service. These codes are stand-alone procedure or service codes, identifying the physician's or provider's professional efforts. In most cases, there are other codes that identify the technical portions of these procedures or services, as well as codes that represent both the professional and technical components, sometimes called global service codes. It is not necessary to report modifier 26 with codes that represent only the professional component of a procedure or service.

CPT code 73110-26 is reported by the radiologist, and the ED physician reports 25530-54.

Example #2:
A patient treated in the ED was sent to the hospital's radiology department for complete knee series. The patient had fallen while roller skating and injured his right knee. Five views were taken of the site, and the patient was returned to the ED for continued treatment. The radiologist read the knee films and dictated a separate report.

CPT code 73564-26 is submitted.

32   MANDATED SERVICES

Services related to mandated consultation and/or related services (e.g., PRO, third-party payer, governmental, legislative, or regulatory requirement) may be identified by adding the modifier 32 to the basic procedure.

Coding Tips
- Modifier 32 is used to indicate mandated health care services.
- Use of modifier 32 on radiology codes is rare. When a consultation is ordered or requested by the payer it would be appropriate to append modifier 32 to radiology services provided during the IME.
- CPT codes for use with modifier 32 are 99201–99499, 00100–01999, 10021–69990, 70010–79999, 80048–89399, and 90281–99600, if appropriate and unless limited by the payer.

Clinical Example
A radiological examination of the upper gastrointestinal tract, without KUB, was ordered by a judge for evidence of ingested plastic drug packets. The subject was apprehended at the airport after arriving from a foreign country.

CPT code 74240-32 is submitted.

50   BILATERAL PROCEDURE

Unless otherwise identified in the listings, bilateral procedures that are performed at the same operative session should be identified by adding the modifier 50 to the appropriate five-digit code.

Using the Modifier Correctly
- For Medicare claims, report the bilateral radiology services with one procedure code appended with modifier 50. This should appear on the CMS-1500 claim form as one-line item, with a unit number of one. However, many Medicare carriers will also accept bilateral procedures reported as two-line items with the right (RT) and left (LT) HCPCS Level II modifiers appended to the respective procedure codes.
- The 50 modifier is not listed in the guidelines of the radiology section of the CPT code book. However, Medicare does accept modifier 50 on select procedures and allows payment at 200 percent when performed bilaterally. Some of these codes are listed below:
    70030, 70120, 70130, 70190, 70332, 70336, 73000, 73010, 73020, 73030, 73040, 73060, 73070, 73080, 73085, 73090, 73092, 73100,

73110, 73115, 73120, 73130, 73140, 73200, 73201, 73202, 73220, 73221, 73525, 73530, 73550, 73560, 73562, 73564, 73580, 73590, 73592, 73600, 73610, 73615, 73620, 73630, 73650, 73660, 73721, 76511, 76512, 76513, 76519, 76529.

Incorrect Use of the Modifier
- Reporting bilateral procedures to Medicare as two line items on the CMS-1500 claim form, appending modifier 50 to the second (bilateral) procedure code, as is correctly done for many other third-party payers. For Medicare claims, however, this is not correct.
- Using modifier 50 on the following radiology codes (they are considered bilateral and the RVUs are already based on the procedure being performed as a bilateral procedure): 71110, 71111, 73050, 73520, 73565, 75662, 75671, 75680, 75803, 75807, 75822, 75833, 75842, 76091, 76094, 76102, 76514, 76516, 76519, and/or 76645.

Coding Tips
- Comparison x-rays are used to assess similarities. When x-rays are performed to compare the corresponding extremity/opposite side in the absence of abnormal signs or symptoms, they are considered screening and are not covered by Medicare. However, there may be times when comparison x-rays of the extremities (73000–73140 and/or 73500–73660) may be considered for coverage. If a beneficiary has an x-ray taken of an extremity which has symptomatology and a definitive diagnosis cannot be made—making it reasonable that a comparison x-ray would assist in the diagnosis—then a comparison x-ray may be eligible for payment. The provider must document the reason for the comparison x-ray. Detailed documentation should be sent with the claim. Either the RT or LT HCPCS Level II modifier is used when these services are performed. Modifier 50 should not be used for comparison x-rays.
- CPT codes for use with modifier 50 are 10021–69990, 70010–79999, and 90281–99600, if appropriate and unless limited by the payer.

Clinical Example
A 16-year-old was skateboarding and suffered a fall onto bilaterally outstretched hands. When he presented to the ED complete x-ray exams were taken of both the right and left wrist. The radiologist read the exam of the left wrist, three views, as not showing a fracture. The right wrist series (four views) were interpreted to have a fracture of the radius at the growth plate.

Report 73110 with modifier 50 or it may be reported as 73110 LT and 73110 RT.

51   MULTIPLE PROCEDURES
When multiple procedures, other than evaluation and management services, are performed at the same session by the same provider, the primary procedure or service may be reported as listed. The additional procedure(s) or service(s) may be identified by appending the modifier 51 to the additional procedure or service code(s). **Note:** This modifier should not be appended to designated add-on codes.

Using the Modifier Correctly
- Modifier 51 is used to indicate that more than one procedure was performed by the same physician on the same patient on the same date of service.
- Report multiple procedures on the same claim using the 51 modifier.

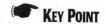

KEY POINT

Modifier 50 should not be used for comparison x-rays. HCPCS Level II modifiers LT and RT should instead be used to identify contralateral films.

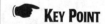

KEY POINT

The 1999 edition of the CPT code book contains two new conventions or symbols: + and ⊘. The + symbol is seen adjacent to CPT codes that represent add-on services, or services commonly carried out in addition to a primary procedure. These add-on codes are, therefore, not to be reported without first reporting the primary procedure code. The symbol ⊘ identifies CPT codes with which the -51 modifier, multiple procedures, should not be reported. For example, CPT code 17004 describes the destruction of benign or premalignant lesions, including local anesthesia, for 15 or more lesions. This code should not be reported with the -51 modifier as the destruction procedures for each of the 15 lesions are inherent in the code's description. Likewise, it should not be reported on the CMS-1500 claim form with a units quantity of 15, as only one unit correctly represents the service.

Incorrect Use of the Modifier

- Code 76390 describes a magnetic resonance spectroscopy for all sites. The CPT manual provides a cross-reference for the use to view the appropriate body site for an MRI. Both codes would be reported if performed and medically necessary. The individual payer should be consulted for instructions on modifier use of 51 as it may not be appropriate to report the MRI studies with modifier 51.
- Using the 51 modifier with add-on secondary codes. These codes are, by description, never used alone, and the assignment of modifier 51 is inappropriate.

Coding Tips

- When multiple procedures, other than E/M services, are performed on the same day or at the same session by the same provider, report the primary procedure or service. The 51 modifier is appended to the appropriate CPT code for the additional service(s) or procedure(s).
- The 51 modifier is not used with add-on codes. Add-on codes are procedures performed in addition to the main procedure. These codes represent procedures that cannot be performed alone. Examples of words to look for as clues to add-on procedures are each additional, list in addition to, and second lesion.
- CPT codes for use with modifier 51 are 00100–01999, 10021–69990, 70010–79999, and 90281–99600, when appropriate unless limited by the payer.

Clinical Example

A patient was involved in a serious motor vehicle accident and brought to the ED. The physician ordered the following films:

- Complete x-ray of the mandible with six views
- X-ray of the left eye for detection of foreign body
- Radiologic exam of the complete spine, survey study, anteroposterior, and lateral views
- Complete skull films

The ED physician would report the above services as follows: 72010-26, 70260-26-51, 70110-26-51, and 70030-26-51.

Although the 51 is added to codes 70260, 70110, and 70030, no reduction in the Medicare allowable should be made. Some payers may prefer the use of modifier 59, distinct procedural service, for the second through fourth radiology services in this example, instead of modifier 51.

52   REDUCED SERVICES

Under certain circumstances a service or procedure is partially reduced or eliminated at the physician's discretion. Under these circumstances the service provided can be identified by its usual procedure number and the addition of the modifier 52, signifying that the service is reduced. This provides a means of reporting reduced services without disturbing the identification of the basic service. **Note:** For hospital outpatient reporting of a previously scheduled procedure/service that is partially reduced or cancelled as a result of extenuating circumstances or those that threaten the well-being of the patient prior to or after administration of anesthesia, see modifiers 73 and 74.

> ### ✓ QUICK TIP
>
> **Hospital ASC and Outpatient Coders**
> Modifier 51 is not applicable in hospital ASC or hospital outpatient facilities in accordance with CPT modifiers approved for ASC outpatient hospital use.

Using the Modifier Correctly
- Modifier 52 is used for reporting services that were partially reduced or eliminated at the physician's election. Documentation should be present in the medical record explaining the circumstances surrounding the reduction in service.
- Modifier 52 is used to indicate that a procedure or service is being performed at a lesser level. A concise statement that describes how the service differs from the normal procedure must be included with the claim.
- When a limited comparative x-ray study is performed (e.g., postreduction radiographs, postintubation, postcatheter placement, etc.), the CPT code for the comprehensive x-ray should be billed with modifier 52, indicating that a reduced level of service was provided.

Incorrect Use of the Modifier
- Using Modifier 52 For Terminated Procedures. This modifier is intended for procedures which accomplished some result, but less than expected for the procedure.
- Using modifier 52 on a time-based code (i.e., critical care, psychotherapy, anesthesia), automated organ or disease panels or codes which specifically state "limited" (e.g., duplex sonography). Check with the carriers to see if they recognize modifier 52 and find out their policy for its use. In some cases, there are alternative choices for coding a lesser service, so the 52 modifier would not be appended.

Coding Tips
- Modifier 52 is used to indicate under certain circumstances, a service or procedure is partially reduced or eliminated at the physician's discretion.
- The 52 modifier is for a reduced service and is not a modifier to be used in situations when the fee is reduced for a patient due to his or her inability to pay the full charges.
- CPT codes for use with modifier 52 are 99201–99499 (except for Medicare), 10021–69990, 70010–79999, 80048–89399, and 90281–99600 (except psychotherapy), when appropriate unless limited by the payer.

Clinical Example
An 88-year-old patient presented to the physician's office with a chief complaint of wrist pain after falling from a chair at home. X-rays (A/P and lateral views of the wrist) revealed a Colles' fracture of the right wrist. The physician performed a closed treatment with manipulation. Following the treatment, the physician ordered a postreduction x-ray.

CPT codes 25605, 73100, 73100-59-52 are used. Use of the 59 modifier in this scenario may not be required by many payers. The 52 modifier is required by Medicare when limited comparative radiographic studies are performed (e.g., postreduction, postintubation, and postcatheter placement radiographs, etc.).

53 DISCONTINUED PROCEDURE
Under certain circumstances, the physician may elect to terminate a surgical or diagnostic procedure. Due to extenuating circumstances or those that threaten the well being of the patient, it may be necessary to indicate that a surgical or diagnostic procedure was started but discontinued. This circumstance may be reported by adding the modifier 53 to the code reported by the physician for the discontinued procedure. **Note:** This modifier is not used to report the elective cancellation of a

QUICK TIP

Hospital ASC and Outpatient Coders

Per Medicare, modifier 52, reduced service, is used in the hospital outpatient department to identify a procedure not requiring anesthesia (meaning general, regional, or local) that was terminated after the patient was prepared for the procedure (including any sedation). Reimbursement for modifier 52 procedures is 50 percent.

When a radiology procedure is reduced, the correct reporting is to code to the extent of the procedure performed. If no code exists for what has been done, report the intended code with modifier 52 appended.

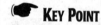

KEY POINT

The *Medicare Carriers Manual* states, in part, that when procedures for which services performed are significantly less than usually required, [these services] may be billed with modifier 52. Radiology procedures reported with this modifier should include the following documentation:
- A concise statement about how the service or procedure differs from the usual
- The operative (or other) report

Claims reported with modifier 52, which do not include documentation that serves to clarify the use of this modifier, will be processed as if there were no modifiers reported.

procedure prior to the patients anesthesia induction and/or surgical preparation in the operating suite. For outpatient hospital/ASC reporting of a previously scheduled procedure/service that is partially reduced or cancelled as a result of extenuating circumstances or those that threaten the well-being of the patient prior to or after administration of anesthesia, see modifiers 73 and 74.

Using the Modifier Correctly

Hospital ASC and Outpatient Coders
Modifier 53 is not applicable in hospital ASC or hospital outpatient facilities in accordance with CPT modifiers approved for ASC outpatient hospital use.

- Modifier 53 is used when a procedure was actually started but had to be discontinued before completion.
- Modifier 53 is used modifier if a radiographic procedure was discontinued due to patient risk.
- If a procedure is discontinued due to uncontrollable bleeding, hypotension, neurologic impairment, or situations that threaten the well-being of the patient, modifier 53 is appended to the surgical or diagnostic procedure code.
- The 53 modifier applies to the physician's office as well. All procedures billed with the 53 modifier may require documentation.

Incorrect Use of the Modifier

- Using modifier 53 to report the elective cancellation of a procedure prior to the patient's anesthesia induction and/or surgical preparation in the operative suite.
- Using modifier 53 when a procedure is prematurely terminated prior to the induction of anesthesia. The correct modifier to report these services is modifier 52.
- Using modifier 53 on an E/M code. Many insurance companies do not recognize modifier 53 on this type of service. Check with individual payers for use of 53 on an E/M code.
- Using modifier 53 on a time-based code (i.e., critical care, psychotherapy, anesthesia), automated organ or disease panels or codes which specifically state "limited" (e.g., duplex sonography). Check with the carriers to see if they recognize modifier 53 and find out their policy for its use. In some cases, there are alternative choices for coding a lesser service, so modifier 53 would not be appended.

Coding Tips

- Modifier 53 is used when under extenuating circumstances or those that threaten the well-being of the patient, the physician may elect to terminate a surgical or diagnostic procedure. This modifier is used when it may be necessary to indicate that a surgical or diagnostic procedure was started but discontinued following anesthesia administration.
- For aborted or discontinued procedures, report the appropriate ICD-9-CM diagnosis code (V64.1, V64.2, or V64.3). Follow individual third-party payer guidelines, as some payers and managed care organizations do not accept V codes.
- CPT codes for use with modifier 53 are 00100–01999, 10021–69990, 70010–79999, 80048–89399, and 90281–99600 unless limited by the payer.

Clinical Example

A patient presented to the hospital radiology department for a urography with KUB, CPT code 74400, for gross hematuria. During the procedure the patient became very anxious and complained of vertigo and nausea. The procedure was discontinued to prevent risk to the patient.

Submit code 74400-26-53.

58 Staged or Related Procedure or Service by the Same Physician During the Postoperative Period

The physician may need to indicate that the performance of a procedure or service during the postoperative period was: a) planned prospectively at the time of the original procedure (staged); b) more extensive than the original procedure; or c) for therapy following a diagnostic surgical procedure. This circumstance may be reported by adding the modifier 58 to the staged or related procedure. **Note:** This modifier is not used to report the treatment of a problem that requires a return to the operating room. See modifier 78.

Using the Modifier Correctly
- Modifier 58 is used only when the second, related procedure or service is performed during the postoperative period.
- Modifier 58 is used for the following:
  —to show a procedure was performed during the postoperative period of another procedure because the subsequent procedure was planned prospectively at the time of an original procedure
  —to show a second procedure was more extensive than the original procedure
  —for therapy following a diagnostic surgical procedure
- A new postoperative period begins when the next procedure in the staged procedure series is billed.
- If more than one physician is involved in a staged procedure, each physician must submit the claim using the 58 and 52 modifier (reduced services). These claims are subject to individual consideration and payment calculation is based on the percentage of the procedure each physician performs.

Incorrect Use of the Modifier
- Using modifier 58 to report the treatment of a problem that requires a return to the operating room. See modifier 78 for that purpose.

Coding Tips
- To report a staged or related procedure add modifier 58. Failure to use this modifier, when appropriate, may result in denial of the subsequent claim.
- Do not use modifier 58 with procedure codes that are described as one or more services. These procedures in the CPT code book are considered multiple sessions or are otherwise defined as including multiple services or events. The Medicare fee schedule RVU was established based on the total procedure. Therefore, separate reimbursement may not be made for each segment of the procedure even if it is for one or more services.
- CPT codes for use with modifier 58 are 10021–69990, 70010–79999, and 90281–99600 unless limited by the payer.

Clinical Example
A patient received clinical brachytherapy by intracavitary application. Treatment was a simple application of one to four ribbons. It was decided prospectively to use a complex application if the initial procedure was not successful.

After 10 days, it was necessary to perform a complex application of 12 ribbons.

CPT code 77761-26 is submitted for the initial procedure and code 77763-26-58 is submitted for the subsequent staged procedure.

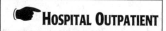

Hospital ASC and Outpatient Coders
Medicare's instructions for modifier 58 in hospital ASC or hospital outpatient facilities include in the definition procedures performed on the same calendar day.

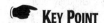

Modifier 58 must be used for purposes of distinguishing procedures performed by the original surgeon or radiologist during the postoperative period of the original (first) procedure, within the constraints of the modifier's definition. These procedures cannot be repeat operations (unless the procedures are more extensive than the original procedure) and cannot be for the treatment of complications requiring a return trip to the operating room.

59   Distinct Procedural Service

Under certain circumstances, the physician may need to indicate that a procedure or service was distinct or independent from other services performed on the same day. Modifier 59 is used to identify procedures/services that are not normally reported together, but are appropriate under the circumstances. This may represent a different session or patient encounter, different procedure or surgery, different site or organ system, separate incision/excision, separate lesion, or separate injury (or area of injury in extensive injuries) not ordinarily encountered or performed on the same day by the same physician. However, when another already established modifier is appropriate it should be used rather than modifier 59. Only if no more descriptive modifier is available, and the use of modifier 59 best explains the circumstances, should modifier 59 be used.

Using the Modifier Correctly

- Modifier 59 is used when billing a combination of codes that would normally not be billed together. This modifier indicates that the ordinarily bundled code represents a service done at a different anatomic site or at a different session on the same date. This may represent:

  —different session or patient encounter

  —different procedure or service on the same day

  —different site or organ system (e.g., a skin graft and an allograft in different locations)

  —separate incision/excision

  —separate lesion (e.g., a biopsy of skin on the neck is performed at the same session as an excision of a 1.0 cm benign lesion of the face)

  —separate injury

- Modifier 59 is used only on the procedure designated as the "distinct procedural service." The physician needs to document that a procedure or service was distinct or separate from other services performed on the same day.

- The medical record documentation must be clear as to the separate and distinct procedure before modifier 59 is appended to a code. This modifier allows the code to bypass edits; therefore, appropriate documentation must be present in the record. **Note:** Medicare uses the Correct Coding Initiative (CCI) screens when editing claims for possible unbundling. Under CCI screens, specific codes have been identified that should not be billed together.

- Modifier 59 is used only if another modifier does not describe the situation more accurately.

Incorrect Use of the Modifier

- Using the 59 modifier on E/M codes.
- Using the modifier 59 as a replacement for modifiers 24, 25, 78, or 79.
- Using modifier 59 when another modifier best describes the distinct service.

Coding Tips

- Modifier 59 is used to indicate that a procedure or service was distinct or independent from other services performed on the same day.
- If there is not a more descriptive modifier available, and the use of modifier 59 best explains the circumstance, then modifier 59 is appended.

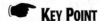

Key Point

Use modifier 59 only when the subsequent procedure occurs on the same date as another procedure by the same provider.

Key Point

Modifier 59 was established (and replaced the HCPCS Level II temporary modifier GB) to demonstrate that multiple yet distinct services were provided to a patient on the same date of service by the same provider. Because distinct procedures or services rendered on the same day by the same physician cannot be easily identified and therefore properly adjudicated by simply listing the CPT procedure codes, modifier 59 assists the third-party payer or Medicare carrier in applying the appropriate reimbursement protocol. If the modifier is not used in these circumstances, a denial of services may ensue, with the explanation of benefits stating, for instance for Medicare claims, "Medicare does not pay for this service because it is part of another service that was performed at the same time."

Quick Tip

Hospital ASC and Outpatient Coders

Modifier 62 is not applicable in hospital ASC or hospital outpatient facilities in accordance with CPT modifiers approved for ASC outpatient hospital use.

- When a procedure or service that is designated as a separate procedure in the CPT manual is carried out independently or considered to be unrelated or distinct from the other services provided at the same session, it may be reported by appending the 59 modifier to the specific separate procedure code to indicate that the procedure is not considered to be a component of another procedure, but instead is a distinct, independent procedure.
- CPT codes for use with 59 modifier are 00100–01999, 10021–69990, 70010–79999, 80048–89399, and 90281–99600, when appropriate unless limited by the payer.

76 Repeat Procedure by Same Physician

The physician may need to indicate that a procedure or service was repeated subsequent to the original procedure or service. This circumstance may be reported by adding the modifier 76 to the repeated procedure/service.

Using the Modifier Correctly
- There are varied policies regarding when and how this modifier is to be applied to a CPT code. Some carriers expect usage on radiology and laboratory services, however, some do not. Check with individual carriers for specific billing instructions.
- Modifier 76 is appended to a code when the same physician repeats the same service, usually on the same day, however, it can be used whenever the circumstances warrant it.
- This modifier is used to indicate that a repeat procedure was necessary and that it does not represent a duplicate bill.

Incorrect Use of the Modifier
- Using modifier 76 to indicate repositioning or replacement 14 days after the initial insertion or replacement of an existing pacemaker or defibrillator. Modifier 76 is not reported with pacemaker or defibrillator codes after 14 days as these are considered new, not repeat, services.

Coding Tips
- Modifier 76 is added to the repeat service to indicate that a procedure or service was repeated subsequent to the original service. An explanation of the medical necessity for the repeat procedure is necessary (e.g., repeat x-ray performed after thoracotomy tube placement).
- Use the appropriate CPT code that describes the type of imaging performed. Codes 78460–78469 describe the characteristics of each type of test, including whether it is a single study or multiple studies. Use the single best code that describes the service. The multiple injection studies may be performed either on one day or as a series of multiple injections on separate days. Do not bill reinjection imaging separately with the same or a different code, same day or different day, or by the same or different provider. Do not append modifier 76 to the CPT code. It is considered to be inclusive in the billing for the entire study. CPT codes 78478 or 78480 describe additions to the above studies and, when performed, can be submitted in addition to the above studies.
- CPT codes for use with modifier 76 unless limited by the payer are 10040–69990, 70010–79999, and 90281–99600, when appropriate.

Quick Tip

Hospital ASC and Outpatient Coders
Medicare's instructions for modifiers 76 and 77 in hospital ASC or hospital outpatient facilities include in the definition procedures "repeated in a separate operative session on the same calendar day." Use modifier 76 for same physician/same day and modifier 77 for another physician/same day. The procedure must be the same procedure.

Clinical Example

Chest x-ray, single view, frontal, performed twice on the same day by the same physician due to aspiration pneumonia.

CPT codes 71010-26 (1 unit) and 71010-26-76 (1 unit) are submitted. This circumstance must be supported by medical necessity documentation sent with the initial claim.

77 REPEAT PROCEDURE BY ANOTHER PHYSICIAN

The physician may need to indicate that a basic procedure or service performed by another physician had to be repeated. This situation may be reported by adding modifier 77 to the repeated procedure/service.

Using the Modifier Correctly

- Modifier 77 is used when an identical service is rendered, usually same day, by a different physician. Check with individual commercial carriers for billing instructions.
- When the identical service is being billed on the same day by a different physician, report the service for example, as follows:
  —physician # 1—Chest, single view, frontal: 71010 (1 unit)
  —physician # 2—Chest, single view, frontal: 71010-77 (1 unit)
- Because a second interpretation and report are unusual in a radiology practice, claims may be audited on a random basis. Documentation which supports the unusual circumstances requiring a second procedure and/or interpretation of findings must be kept in the patient's file and be available upon request of the carrier. Check with the local carrier for its policy regarding second procedures, interpretations and reports.

Incorrect Use of the Modifier

- Using modifier 77 to indicate repositioning or replacement 14 days after the initial insertion or replacement of an existing pacemaker or defibrillator. Modifier 77 is not reported with pacemaker or defibrillator codes after 14 days as these are considered new, not repeat services.

Coding Tips

- Modifier 77 is added to the repeated service to indicate that a basic procedure or service performed by another physician needed to be repeated by a different physician. An explanation of the medical necessity for the repeat service is necessary.
- Modifier 77 is used to show the third-party payer that the services were actually rendered again on the same date. This will help them to distinguish claim submissions from those that are inadvertently duplicated billings.
- Modifier 77 does not guarantee reimbursement of repeated services as other third-party payer regulations (such as medical necessity) are still applicable.
- CPT codes for use with modifier 77 unless limited by the payer are 10021–69990, 70010–79999, and 90281–99600, when appropriate.

Clinical Example

An internist ordered a radiological examination of the chest, complete, minimum of four views on a patient with a chronic cough with sputum production. The patient reports chest tightness recently and inability to take a deep breath. Patient has

---

> ### ✓ QUICK TIP
>
> For services furnished on or after January 1, 1996, the policy for payments for the interpretation of an x-ray furnished to a Medicare patient in an ED by a hospital-based radiologist has been changed. Payment for the interpretation will now be allowed to either the specialist or the treating physician. As part of the revised policy, CMS specified that the professional component of a diagnostic procedure furnished to a beneficiary in a hospital must include an interpretation and written report for inclusion in the beneficiary's medical record maintained by the hospital. Under the revised policy, CMS has made a distinction between an interpretation and report of an x-ray and a review of the procedure. A claim for the professional component of x-ray services based on a review of the findings of radiology procedures without a complete, written report does not meet the conditions for separate payment of these services. An interpretation and report should address the findings, relevant clinical issues, and comparative data (when available) such as prior x-rays. To allow for the unusual need for a second official interpretation and report, report the medically necessity of the second interpretation with modifier 77, indicating that a second procedure was required. When this modifier is attached, both claims may be paid.

smoked three packs/day for 40 years. The x-rays were positive for a suspicious mass in the right lung and shadows in the left lung.

The internist coordinated care with a local pulmonologist and the patient was sent on the same day for an evaluation. The pulmonologist repeated the chest x-rays with a darker density, in order to see the mass.

CPT code 71030-77 is submitted by the pulmonologist.

99   Multiple Modifiers

Under certain circumstances two or more modifiers may be necessary to completely delineate a service. In such situations modifier 99 should be added to the basic procedure, and the other applicable modifiers may be listed as part of the description of the service.

Using the Modifier Correctly
- The modifier 99 is placed after a selected CPT code to illustrate to the payer that multiple modifiers apply to the service(s). Use modifier 99 on the basic service. Enter on the CMS-1500 claim form all applicable additional modifiers in item 19. If modifier 99 is entered on multiple line items, all applicable modifiers for each line item containing a 99 modifier should be listed as follows: 1 = (mod), where the numeral "1" represents the specific line item and mod represents all modifiers applicable to the referenced line item. For electronic submissions, the additional modifiers should be listed in the extra narrative field, record HAO, field 05.0, positions 40 through 320. If the individual modifiers are not identified, the claim may be denied.

Incorrect Use of the Modifier
- Applying modifier 99 to a code with no additional or just one additional modifier.

Coding Tips
- Modifier 99 is added to the basic service when more than two modifiers are needed to describe a service. The additional modifiers should be included with the claim (item 19 on paper claim submissions, or the appropriate message in the freeform area on electronic submissions).
- Before using modifier 99, check with third-party payers regarding their rules for its use.
- CPT codes for use with modifier 99 are 10021–69990, 70010–79999, and 90281–99600, when appropriate unless limited by the payer.

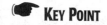

Key Point

Submitting 99 by Electronic Claims

When submitting modifier 99, multiple modifiers, by electronic claims, many third-party payers, including some Medicare carriers, require the modifier 99 in the first modifier field, the second modifier in the second modifier field, and the remaining modifiers in the narrative (HAO) record.

When submitting only two modifiers or less and, therefore, not reporting the modifier 99, continue to use only the first and second modifier fields.

Chapter 5: Pathology and Laboratory

22   UNUSUAL PROCEDURAL SERVICES

When the service(s) provided is greater than that usually required for the listed procedure, it may be identified by adding modifier 22 to the usual procedure number. A report may also be appropriate. **Note:** This modifier is not to be used to report procedure(s) complicated by adhesion formation, scarring, and/or alteration of normal landmarks due to late effects of prior surgery, irradiation, infection, very low weight (i.e., neonates and infants less than 4 kg), or trauma.

Using the Modifier Correctly
- Modifier 22 is used to the basic CPT code book procedure code when the service(s) provided is greater than usually required for the listed procedure. Use of modifier 22 on services requires individual consideration of the claim(s).
- Modifier 22 is used to identify an increment of work that is infrequently encountered with a particular procedure and is not described by another code.
- The frequent use of modifier 22 has prompted many carriers to ignore it. When using modifier 22, the claim must be accompanied by documentation and a cover letter explaining the unusual circumstances. Documentation includes, but is not limited to, descriptive statements identifying the unusual circumstances, operative reports (state the usual time for performing the procedure and the prolonged time due to any complications), pathology reports, progress notes, office notes, etc.

Incorrect Use of the Modifier
- Appending this modifier to a code without justification in the medical record of an unusual occurrence. Because of its overuse, many payers do not acknowledge this modifier.
- Using this modifier on a routine basis. To do so would most certainly flag the claim and may result in an audit.
- Using modifier 22 to indicate a procedure was performed by a specialist. Specialty designation does not warrant use of modifier 22.

Coding Tips
- Using modifier 22 identifies the service as one requiring individual consideration and manual review.
- Overuse of modifier 22 could trigger a carrier audit. Carriers monitor the use of this modifier very carefully. Make sure that modifier 22 is used only when sufficient documentation is present in the medical record.
- A Medicare claim submitted with modifier 22 is forwarded to the carrier medical review staff for review and pricing. With sufficient documentation of medical necessity increased payment may result.

QUICK TIP

Hospital ASC and Outpatient Coders
Modifier 22 is not applicable in hospital ASC or hospital outpatient facilities in accordance with CPT modifiers approved for ambulatory surgery center (ASC) outpatient hospital use.

KEY POINT

Claims submitted to Medicare, Medicaid, and other third-party payers containing modifier 22 for unusual procedural services that do not have attached supporting documentation that demonstrates the unusual distinction of the services will generally be processed as if the procedure codes were not appended with the modifier. Some third-party payers might suspend the claims and request additional information from the respective providers, but this is the exception rather than the rule.

KEY POINT

Do not bombard the Medicare carrier or other third-party payer with unnecessary documentation. All attachments to the claim for justification of the unusual services should explain the unusual circumstances in a concise, clear manner. The information for the justification of unusual services should be easy to locate within the attached documentation. Highlight this information, if necessary, to facilitate the medical reviewer's access to the pertinent supporting data.

- A claim with modifier 22 will be processed on a by-report basis and will cause the claim processing to be delayed. In these cases, Medicare will consider the unusual nature of the service and, if they believe a charge above the fee schedule is justified, will approve an amount that recognizes the additional services. This, in effect, becomes a higher-than-usual fee schedule amount for the service. The approved amount (or higher fee schedule amount) is the basis of the limiting charge calculation for modifier 22 services. Therefore, if the billed amount exceeds Medicare's approved amount by more than 15 percent, an adjustment must be made or a refund to the patient must be made in order to meet the limiting charge requirements of the law. Because the exact limiting charge in these cases is not known until the claims payment decision is made, Medicare would not consider these cases as knowing or willful violations, provided the physician made the appropriate adjustments or refunds.
- Use of this modifier to report laboratory services is rare. Check with payers for individual policy.
- CPT codes for use with modifier 22 are 00100–01999, 10021–69990, 70010–79999, 80048–89399, when appropriate, and 90281–99600 unless limited by the payer.

26   PROFESSIONAL COMPONENT

Certain procedures are a combination of a physician component and a technical component. When the physician component is reported separately, the service may be identified by adding the modifier 26 to the usual procedure number.

Using the Modifier Correctly

- Modifier 26 is appended to the laboratory procedure code to report that only the professional component portion of the procedure is being reported.
- Modifier 26 is used in those instances during which a physician provides the interpretation of the diagnostic test/study performed. The interpretation of the diagnostic test/study has to be separate, distinct, identifiable, written and signed.

Incorrect Use of the Modifier

- Using modifiers 26 and TC for technical components (except for purchased diagnostic tests) when a diagnostic test is performed globally (both components are performed by the same provider). When a global service is performed, it should be coded as a single procedure without modifiers. The payment for the global service will reflect the allowances for both components.
- Using the 26 modifier for a reread of results of an interpretation initially provided by another physician.
- Using both modifier 26 indicating that only the professional portion of the service was provided and modifier 52 for reduced service. It is not necessary to use 52, since the professional modifier already indicates that only a portion of the complete service was performed.
- Using modifier 26 on codes that are technical component only codes.

Coding Tips

- Certain procedures are a combination of a physician component and a technical component. To report the physician component separately, add modifier 26 to the procedure code.

KEY POINT

There are certain procedure codes that describe and represent only the professional component portion of a procedure or service. These codes are stand-alone procedure or service codes, identifying the physician's or provider's professional efforts. In most cases, there are other procedure or service codes that identify the technical component only, and codes that represent both the professional and technical components as complete procedures or services called global service codes. It is not necessary to report modifier 26 with codes that aptly describe and represent only the professional component of a procedure or service.

- In order to use the professional component modifier 26, the provider must prepare a written report that includes findings, relevant clinical issues, and if appropriate, comparative data. This report must be available if requested by the carrier. A review of the diagnostic procedure findings, without a written report similar to that which would be prepared by a specialist in the field, does not meet the conditions for use of this modifier. If a postpayment review of the medical record reveals that no separate, written report exists, overpayment recoveries may be sought.
- There are procedure codes that identify the professional component of clinical laboratory procedures for which separate payment may be made only if the physician interprets an abnormal smear for the patient. This applies only to the following procedure codes: P3001-26, 85060, 85097, 88104, 88106, 88107, 88108, 88125, 88160, 88161, 88162, 88172, 88173, 88180, 88182, and 88141.
- CPT codes for use with modifier 26 are 10021–69990, 70010–79999, 80048–89399, and 90281–99600 unless limited by the payer.

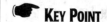

KEY POINT

In order to use a PC modifier 26, the provider must prepare a written report that includes findings, relevant clinical issues, and if appropriate, comparative data.

32   MANDATED SERVICES

Services related to mandated consultation and/or related services (e.g., QIO, third-party payer, governmental, legislative, or regulatory requirement) may be identified by adding the modifier 32 to the basic procedure.

Using the Modifier Correctly
- Use modifier 32 when the physician is aware of third-party payer involvement. Legal entities such as the court system can mandate services as well.
- Documentation must support the use of modifier 32 for a mandated service and it must support medical necessity. Who and why must be clearly written in the medical record.

Incorrect Use of the Modifier
- Lack of understanding as to the intent of this modifier may lead to inappropriate assignment. Do not use this modifier when a patient or family member requests a second opinion.

Coding Tips
- Modifier 32 is used to indicate mandated health care services.
- CPT codes for use with modifier 32, unless limited by the payer, are 99201–99499, 00100–01999, 10021–69990, 70010–79999, 80048–89399, and 90281–99600.

Clinical Example
Specimen is collected for a mandated HTLV antibody test (Western Blot). The Warden mandated the service because the patient (a prisoner) bit another prisoner during a fight. Submit CPT code 86689-32.

52   REDUCED SERVICES

Under certain circumstances a service or procedure is partially reduced or eliminated at the physician's discretion. Under these circumstances the service provided can be identified by its usual procedure number and the addition of the modifier 52, signifying that the service is reduced. This provides a means of reporting reduced services without disturbing the identification of the basic service. **Note:** For hospital

Ingenix Coding Lab: Understanding Modifiers

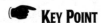

Quick Tip

Hospital ASC and Outpatient Coders

Per Medicare, modifier 52, reduced service, is used in the hospital outpatient department to identify a procedure not requiring anesthesia (meaning general, regional, or local) that was terminated after the patient was prepared for the procedure (including any sedation). Reimbursement for modifier 52 procedures is 50 percent.

Key Point

The *Medicare Carriers Manual* states, in part, that when procedures for which services performed are significantly less than usually required, [these services] may be billed with modifier 52. Laboratory procedures reported with this modifier should include the following documentation:

- A concise statement about how the service or procedure differs from the usual
- The operative report

Claims reported with modifier 52 that do not include the required documentation will be processed as if there were no modifiers reported.

Quick Tip

Hospital ASC and Outpatient Coders

Modifier 53 is not applicable in hospital ASC or hospital outpatient facilities in accordance with CPT modifiers approved for ASC outpatient hospital use.

outpatient reporting of a previously scheduled procedure/service that is partially reduced or cancelled as a result of extenuating circumstances or those that threaten the well-being of the patient prior to or after administration of anesthesia, see modifiers 73 and 74.

Using the Modifier Correctly

- Modifier 52 is used for reporting services that were partially reduced or eliminated at the physician's election. Documentation should be present in the medical record explaining the reduction.
- Modifier 52 is used to indicate that a procedure is being performed at a lesser level. A concise statement that describes how the service differs from the normal procedure must be included with the claim.

Incorrect Use of the Modifier

- Using modifier 52 on a time-based code (i.e., critical care, psychotherapy, anesthesia), automated organ or disease panels or codes which specifically state "limited" (e.g., duplex sonography). Check with your carriers to see if they recognize modifier 52 and find out their policy for its use. In some cases, there are alternative choices for coding a lesser service, so the 52 modifier would not be appended.
- Using modifier 52 if the procedure was terminated either for nonmedical or medical reasons before the ambulatory surgery center (ASC) has expended substantial resources.

Coding Tips

- Use modifier 52 to indicate under certain circumstances, a service or procedure is partially reduced or eliminated at the physician's discretion.
- Modifier 52 is for a reduced service and is not a modifier to be used just because the fee is reduced due to a patient's inability to pay.
- CPT codes for use with modifier 52 are 99201–99499 (except for Medicare), 10021–69990, 70010–79999, 80048–89399, and 90281–99600 (except psychotherapy), when appropriate unless limited by the payer.

Clinical Example

A patient presents to the lab with written orders for a glucose tolerance test (GTT), three specimens (includes glucose), CPT code 82951. Following the second specimen and before the third can be obtained the patient is paged by her infant's daycare provider, and she must leave immediately. The test is not completed.

53   Discontinued Procedure

Under certain circumstances, the physician may elect to terminate a surgical or diagnostic procedure. Due to extenuating circumstances or those that threaten the well-being of the patient, it may be necessary to indicate that a surgical or diagnostic procedure was started but discontinued. This circumstance may be reported by adding the modifier 53 to the code reported by the physician for the discontinued procedure. **Note:** This modifier is not used to report the elective cancellation of a procedure prior to the patient's anesthesia induction and/or surgical preparation in the operating suite. For outpatient hospital/ASC reporting of a previously scheduled procedure/service that is partially reduced or cancelled as a result of extenuating circumstances or those that threaten the well-being of the patient prior to or after administration of anesthesia, see modifiers 73 and 74.

Using the Modifier Correctly
- Modifier 53 is used when a procedure was actually started but had to be discontinued before completion.
- All procedures billed with the 53 modifier may require documentation.

Incorrect Use of the Modifier
- Using modifier 53 when a procedure is prematurely terminated prior to the induction of anesthesia. The correct modifier to report these services is modifier 52.

Coding Tips
- Modifier 53 is used when under extenuating circumstances or those that threaten the well-being of the patient, the physician may elect to terminate a surgical or diagnostic procedure. Use this modifier when it may be necessary to indicate that a surgical or diagnostic procedure was started but was discontinued.
- For aborted or discontinued procedures, report the appropriate ICD-9-CM diagnosis code (V64.1, V64.2, or V64.3).
- Follow individual third-party payer guidelines, as some payers and managed care organizations do not accept V codes.
- CPT codes for use with modifier 53 are 00100–01999, 10021–69990, 70010–79999, 80048–89399, and 90281–99600 unless limited by the payer.

59 DISTINCT PROCEDURAL SERVICE

Under certain circumstances, the physician may need to indicate that a procedure or service was distinct or independent from other services performed on the same day. Modifier 59 is used to identify procedures/services that are not normally reported together, but are appropriate under the circumstances. This may represent a different session or patient encounter, different procedure or surgery, different site or organ system, separate incision/excision, separate lesion, or injury (or area of injury in extensive injuries) not ordinarily encountered or performed on the same day by the same physician. However, when another already established modifier is appropriate it should be used rather than modifier 59. Only if no more descriptive modifier is available, and the use of modifier 59 best explains the circumstances, should modifier 59 be used.

Using the Modifier Correctly
- Modifier 59 is used when a billing a combination of codes that would normally not be billed together. This modifier indicates that the ordinarily bundled code represents a service done at a different anatomic site or at a different session on the same date. This may represent:
  —different session or patient encounter

  —different procedure or service/same day

  —different site or organ system (e.g., a skin graft and an allograft in different locations)

  —separate incision/excision

  —separate lesion (e.g., a biopsy of skin on the neck is performed at the same session as an excision of a 1.0 cm benign lesion of the face)

  —separate injury

 KEY POINT

Modifier 59 was established (and replaced the HCPCS Level II temporary modifier GB) to demonstrate that multiple yet distinct services were provided to a patient on the same date of service by the same provider. Because distinct procedures or services rendered on the same day by the same physician cannot be easily identified and therefore properly adjudicated by simply listing the CPT procedure codes, modifier 59 assists the third-party payer or Medicare carrier in applying the appropriate reimbursement protocol. If the modifier is not used in these circumstances, a denial of services may ensue, with the explanation of benefits stating, for instance for Medicare claims, "Medicare does not pay for this service because it is part of another service that was performed at the same time."

 KEY POINT

Use modifier 59 only when the subsequent procedure occurs on the same date as another procedure by the same provider.

- Modifier 59 is used only on the procedure designated as the distinct procedural service. The physician needs to document that a procedure or service was distinct or separate from other services performed on the same day.
- The medical record documentation must be clear as to the separate distinct procedure before appending modifier 59 to a code. This modifier allows the code to bypass edits, so appropriate documentation must be present in the record. **Note:** Medicare uses CCI edits when processing claims. Under CCI edits, specific codes have been identified that should not be billed together.
- Modifier 59 is used only if another modifier does not describe the situation more accurately.
- When cytopathology codes are billed, the appropriate CPT code to report is that which describes, to the highest level of specificity, the services rendered. Accordingly, for a given specimen, only one code from a family of progressive codes (e.g., codes 88104–88108, 88150–88155, 88160–88162). If multiple services on different specimens are billed, use the 59 modifier to indicate that different levels of service were provided for different specimens. This should be reflected in the cytopathology reports.
- When it is medically necessary to evaluate both bone structure and bone marrow, and both evaluations are provided with one biopsy, then only one CPT code (38221 or 20220–20251) can be billed. If two separate biopsies are necessary, then report both biopsies using the 59 modifier on the second code. Report pathological interpretations codes 88300–88309 individually for multiple separately submitted specimens. If only one specimen is submitted, bill only one code regardless of whether the report includes evaluation of both bone structure and bone marrow morphology or not.
- When multiple approaches are taken to obtain a tissue sample (cytological or surgical), bill the most invasive procedure performed at the same session/site in order to obtain a specimen. For example, if a fine-needle aspiration (CPT codes 88172–88173) is attempted and is unsuccessful and the same physician proceeds to obtain a core biopsy using a cutting needle, and ultimately, finds it necessary to perform an open biopsy, all occurring at the same session, then only bill the open biopsy. In the event different lesions are biopsied using different methodologies, even at the same session, use the 59 modifier. If different biopsy procedures are necessary for different reasons (i.e., fine needle aspiration for diagnosis and needle biopsy for receptors in breast carcinoma), then bill both procedures.

Incorrect Use of the Modifier
- Using the 59 modifier with E/M codes.
- Using modifier 59 when another modifier best describes the distinct service.

Coding Tips
- Modifier 59 is used to indicate that a procedure or service was distinct or independent from other services performed on the same day.
- If there is not a more descriptive modifier available, and the use of modifier 59 best explains the circumstance, then modifier 59 is appended.
- CPT codes for use with 59 modifier are 00100–01999, 10021–69990, 70010–79999, 80048–89399, and 90281–99600, when appropriate unless limited by the payer.

©2003 Ingenix, Inc.
CPT only ©2003 American Medical Association. All Rights Reserved.

Clinical Example

During a patient session, different lesions are biopsied using different methodologies (e.g., fine needle aspiration for diagnosis followed by needle biopsy for receptors in breast carcinoma).

CPT codes 19100 and 88170-59 are submitted.

90   REFERENCE (OUTSIDE) LABORATORY

When laboratory procedures are performed by a party other than the treating or reporting physician, the procedures may be identified by adding the modifier 90 to the usual procedure number.

Coding Tips

- Modifier 90 is added to the usual procedure code when laboratory procedures are performed by a party other than the treating or reporting physician.
- By appending the 90 modifier to the laboratory codes, the physician office is indicating the laboratory procedures were actually performed by an outside laboratory. Medicare does not allow the physician office to bill for the laboratory tests unless it actually performs the tests. If the laboratory performs the tests, the laboratory must bill for these services.
- CPT codes for use with modifier 90 are typically only those found in the range of 80048–89399, unless other CPT codes appended with this modifier are accepted by the individual third-party payer.

Clinical Example

A non-Medicare patient presents for his routine examination and his physician orders a complete blood count (CBC). The physician has contracted with a laboratory to perform the testing, as he has found that performing his own laboratory tests is not cost effective. The medical assistant draws the blood for a CBC as ordered by the physician for a routine medical exam, and sends it to the laboratory. The billing staff will need to indicate that the laboratory test was performed by an outside laboratory (85024-90) as the physician will bill the patient for the service and the laboratory, in turn, will bill the physician.

91   REPEAT CLINICAL DIAGNOSTIC LABORATORY TEST

In the course of treatment of the patient, it may be necessary to repeat the same laboratory test on the same day to obtain subsequent (multiple) test results. Under these circumstances, the laboratory test performed can be identified by its usual procedure number and the addition of the modifier 91. **Note:** This modifier may not be used when tests are rerun to confirm initial results; due to testing problems with specimens or equipment; or for any other reason when a normal, one-time, reportable result is all that is required. This modifier may not be used when other code(s) describe a series of test results (e.g., glucose tolerance tests, evocative/suppression testing). This modifier may only be used for laboratory test(s) performed more than once on the same day on the same patient.

Coding Tips

- Modifier 91 is added to the procedure code(s) that represent repeat laboratory tests or studies performed on the same day on the same patient.

Hospital ASC and Outpatient Coders
Modifier 90 is not applicable in hospital ASC or hospital outpatient facilities in accordance with CPT modifiers approved for ASC outpatient hospital use.

Referring physicians are required to provide diagnostic information to the testing entity at the time the test is ordered. All diagnostic tests must be ordered by the physician treating the beneficiary. An order may include the following forms of communication:

- A written document signed by the treating physician/practitioner, which is hand-delivered, mailed or faxed to the testing facility
- A telephone call by the treating physician/practitioner or his/her office to the testing facility
- An electronic mail by the treating physician/practitioner or his/her office to the testing facility

Note: If the order is communicated via telephone, both the treating physician/practitioner or his/her office and the testing facility must document the telephone call in their respective copies of the beneficiary's records.

Ingenix Coding Lab: Understanding Modifiers

- Add modifier 91 only when additional test results are to be obtained subsequent to the administration or performance of the same test(s) on the same day.
- Modifier 91 is not used when laboratory tests or studies are simply rerun because of specimen or equipment error or malfunction.
- Modifier 91 should not be reported when the basic procedure code(s) indicate that a series of test results are to be obtained, such as CPT code 82951, glucose; tolerance test (GTT), three specimens (includes glucose).

Example #1:

A patient with a history of unstable non-insulin-dependent diabetes mellitus (NIDDM) undergoes an initial glucometry test in the physician's office. The results of this test reveal an extraordinarily high circulating glucose, and confirm the suspicion of uncontrolled NIDDM. The patient is administered 1000 mg of Glucophage, p.o., in the office and is observed for some time. A repeat glucometry reading is obtained, with a satisfactory decline in the circulating glucose noted.

Note: The physician's office holds a CLIA-waived registration for laboratory testing.

Chapter 6: Medicine

22   Unusual Services

When the service(s) provided is greater than that usually required for the listed procedure, it may be identified by adding modifier 22 to the usual procedure number. A report may also be appropriate. **Note:** This modifier is not to be used to report procedure(s) complicated by adhesion formation, scarring, and/or alteration of normal landmarks due to late effects of prior surgery, irradiation, infection, very low weight (i.e., neonates and infants less than 4 kg), or trauma.

Using the Modifier Correctly

- Modifier 22 is appended to the basic CPT procedure code when the service(s) provided is greater than usually required for the listed procedure. Use of modifier 22 on services requires individual claim consideration.
- Modifier 22 is used to identify an increment of work that is infrequently encountered with a particular procedure and is not described by another code.
- The frequent reporting of modifier 22 has prompted many carriers to ignore it. When using modifier 22, the claim must be accompanied by documentation and a cover letter explaining the unusual circumstances. Documentation includes, but is not limited to, descriptive statements identifying the unusual circumstances, operative reports (state the usual time for performing the procedure and the prolonged time due to complication), pathology reports, progress notes, office notes, etc. Some words that indicate unusual circumstances would be difficult, increased risk, extended, etc. If a slight extension of the procedure was necessary (e.g., a procedure is extended by 15–20 minutes), this minimal prolonged time does not validate the use of modifier 22.
- Surgical or medical procedures that require additional physician "work" due to complications or medical emergencies may warrant the use of modifier 22.
- Modifier 22 is used with the following codes in the medicine section of the CPT manual, when an unusual circumstance is well-documented. The following list is not all-inclusive:
  —biofeedback procedure codes 90901 and 90911
  —hemodialysis procedure codes 90935, 90937, and 90939
  —peritoneal dialysis procedure codes 90945, 90947, and 90997
  —gastroenterology procedure codes 91000–91299
  —nasopharyngoscopy procedure codes 92502 and 92511
  —cardiovascular procedure codes 92950–92998
  —cardiac catheterization procedure codes 93501–93581
  —intracardiac electrophysiological procedure codes 93600–93660

Incorrect Use of the Modifier

- Appending this modifier to a code without justification in the medical record of an unusual occurrence. Because of its overuse, many payers do not acknowledge this modifier.
- Using this modifier on a routine basis. To do so would most certainly flag the claim and may result in an audit.

Quick Tip

Hospital ASC and Outpatient Coders
Modifier 22 is not applicable in hospital ASC or hospital outpatient facilities in accordance with CPT modifiers approved for ambulatory surgery center (ASC) outpatient hospital use.

Key Point

Claims submitted to Medicare, Medicaid, and other third-party payers containing modifier 22 for unusual procedural services that do not have attached supporting documentation that demonstrates the unusual distinction of the services will generally be processed as if the procedure codes were not appended with the modifier. Some third-party payers might suspend the claims and request additional information from the respective providers, but this is the exception rather than the rule.

Ingenix Coding Lab: Understanding Modifiers

- Using modifier 22 to indicate a procedure performed by a specialist. Specialty designation does not warrant use of the 22 modifier.
- Appending modifier 22 to codes 93620–93622 to describe successful or unsuccessful arrhythmia induction. Attempted arrhythmia induction is an inclusive component of CPT codes 93620–93622. Failure to induce the suspected arrhythmia does not alter the reporting of these codes. The code description includes specific nomenclature clarifying the inclusion or exclusion of arrhythmia induction or attempted induction.

Coding Tips

- Using modifier 22 identifies the service as one requiring individual consideration and manual review.
- Overuse of modifier 22 could trigger a carrier audit. Carriers monitor the use of this modifier very carefully. Modifier 22 is used only when sufficient documentation is present in the medical record.
- A Medicare claim submitted with modifier 22 is forwarded to the carrier medical review staff for review and pricing. With sufficient documentation of medical necessity, increased payment may result.
- Modifier 22 is used on all procedure codes with a Medicare global period of zero, 10, or 90 days when unusual circumstances warrant consideration of payment in excess of the fee schedule allowance. This includes services that have a global period but are not surgical services.
- For a nonparticipating physician, the limiting charge provisions (see next bullet) apply to services that are billed with modifier 22 and to all claims submitted to Medicare as a secondary payer, if the services billed are those on the physician fee schedule and subject to charge limits. In all cases, the limiting charge cannot exceed a percentage of the allowable amount. This is the case even in instances where the allowance amount will not be known until the claims are individually priced.
- A claim with modifier 22 will be processed on a by-report basis and will cause the claim processing to be delayed. In these cases, Medicare will consider the unusual nature of the service and, if it believes a charge above the fee schedule is justified, will approve an amount that recognizes the additional service. This in effect becomes a higher-than-usual fee schedule amount for the service. The approved amount (or higher fee schedule amount) is the basis of the limiting charge calculation for modifier 22 services. Therefore, if the billed amount exceeds Medicare's approved amount by more than 15 percent, you must make an adjustment or a refund to the patient in order to meet the limiting charge requirements of the law. Since the exact limiting charge on these cases is not known until the claims payment decision is made, Medicare would not consider these cases as knowing or willful violations, provided the physician made the appropriate adjustments or refunds.
- CPT codes for use with modifier 22 are 00100–01999, 10021–69990, 70010–79999, 80048–89399, and 90281–99600 unless limited by the payer.

> **KEY POINT**
>
> Do not bombard the Medicare carrier or other third-party payer with unnecessary documentation. All attachments to the claim for justification of the unusual services should explain the unusual circumstances in a concise, clear manner. The information for the justification of unusual services should be easy to locate within the attached documentation. Highlight this information, if necessary, to facilitate the medical reviewer's access to the pertinent supporting data.

26 Professional Component

Certain procedures are a combination of a physician component and a technical component. When the physician component is reported separately, the service may be identified by adding modifier 26 to the usual procedure number.

> **KEY POINT**
>
> In order to use a PC modifier 26, the provider must prepare a written report that includes findings, relevant clinical issues, and if appropriate, comparative data.

Using the Modifier Correctly
- Append modifier 26 to the procedure code to report only the professional component.
- Modifier 26 is used in those instances in which a physician is providing the interpretation of the diagnostic test/study performed. The interpretation of the diagnostic test/study has to be separate, distinct, identifiable, written, and signed.

Incorrect Use of the Modifier
- Using modifiers 26 and TC for technical component (except for purchased diagnostic tests) when a diagnostic test or radiology service is performed globally (both components are performed by the same provider). When a global service is performed, it should be coded as a single procedure without modifiers. The payment for the global service will reflect the allowances for both components.
- Using modifier 26 on a technical component only procedure code.
- Using modifier 26 for a reread of results of an interpretation initially provided by another physician.
- Using both modifier 26 indicating that only the professional portion of the service was provided and modifier 52 for reduced services. It is not necessary to use 52 because the professional component modifier already indicates that only a portion of the complete service was provided or performed.

Coding Tips
- Certain procedures are a combination of a physician component and a technical component. To report the physician component (professional) separately, add modifier 26 to the procedure code.
- In order to use the professional component modifier 26, the provider must prepare a written report that includes findings, relevant clinical issues and, if appropriate, comparative data. This report must be available if requested by the carrier. A review of the diagnostic procedure findings, without a written report similar to that which would be prepared by a specialist in the field, does not meet the conditions for modifier use. The review of the findings, usually documented in the medical record or on a machine-generated report as "fx-tibia" or "EKG-WNL" does not suffice as a separately identifiable and, therefore, payable interpretation and report. This simplistic review of the findings should be bundled into any E/M code billed for that date. If a postpayment review of the medical record reveals that no separate, written interpretation and report exists, overpayment recoveries may be sought.
- CPT codes for use with modifier 26 are 10021–69990, 70010–79999, 80048–89399, and 90281–99600 unless limited by the payer.

Clinical Example
A patient presented to the outpatient clinic for a bronchospasm evaluation. The patient has a positive history for heavy smoking (two packs/day/30 years).

The patient has been experiencing a heavy cough with sputum production. The internist performed a spirometry with before and after bronchodilation.

CPT code 94060-26 is submitted.

KEY POINT

There are certain procedure codes that describe and represent only the professional component portion of a procedure or service. These codes are stand-alone procedure or service codes, identifying the physician's or provider's professional efforts. In most cases, there are other procedure or service codes that identify the technical component only, and codes that represent both the professional and technical components as complete procedures or services (called global service codes). It is not necessary to report modifier 26 with codes that aptly describe and represent only the professional component of a procedure or service.

32 MANDATED SERVICES

Services related to mandated consultation and/or related services (e.g., QIO, third-party payer, governmental, legislative, or regulatory requirement) may be identified by adding the modifier 32 to the basic procedure.

Using the Modifier Correctly

- Modifier 32 is used when the physician is aware of third-party involvement regarding mandated services.
- Documentation must support the use of modifier 32 for a mandated service and it must support medical necessity. Who and why must be clearly written in the medical record.
- Modifier 32 is considered informational and, when used, many insurers allow 100 percent reimbursement without a deductible or copay. However, modifier 32 has no effect on Medicare payment.

Incorrect Use of the Modifier

- Lack of understanding as to the intent of this modifier may lead to inappropriate assignment. Do not use this modifier when a patient or family member requests a second opinion.

Coding Tips

- Modifier 32 is used to indicate mandated health care services.
- A common situation where one would see this modifier used would be in a workers' compensation case. Oftentimes, the insurance company paying for the services will ask the patient to see a different doctor for another opinion.
- CPT codes for use with modifier 32 (unless limited by the payer) are 99201–99499, 00100–01999, 10021–69990, 70010–79999, 80048–89399, and 90281–99600.

Clinical Example

A patient was sent to the psychiatrist for a court-ordered psychiatric evaluation. The patient was due to stand trial for repeated acts of violence. The psychiatrist conducted a psychiatric diagnostic interview examination, lasting two hours.

CPT code 90801 32 is submitted. The 32 modifier illustrates a mandated service.

50 BILATERAL PROCEDURE

Unless otherwise identified in the listings, bilateral procedures that are performed at the same operative session should be identified by adding the modifier 50 to the appropriate five-digit code.

Coding Tips

- Medicare does accept modifier 50 on select medicine procedures and allows payment at 200 percent when performed bilaterally. Check the MPFSDB to verify eligibility of modifier 50.
- Medicare considers the following ophthalmologic codes bilateral. Therefore, do not use modifier 50 on 92020, 92060, 92065, 92081, 92082, 92083, 92100, 92120, 92130, 92140, 92250, 92260, 92265, 92275, 92286, 92287, 92312, 92316, 92353, 92354, 92355, 92358, 92371, 92392, 92395, or 92396. If one of the above codes is performed unilaterally, bill the code with modifier LT or RT to indicate that one eye was treated. Medicare will pay for only one eye (i.e., 50 percent of the allowable for the code).

©2003 Ingenix, Inc.
CPT only ©2003 American Medical Association. All Rights Reserved.

The accepted application of modifier 50 for many third-party payers (except for Medicare) is shown below: the bilateral (additional) procedure is identified on the CMS-1500 by reporting modifier 50 with the appropriate procedure code. The first procedure is reported without the addition of the 50 modifier. For instance:

92225 Ophthalmoscopy, extended, with retinal drawing (e.g., for retinal detachment, melanoma), with interpretation and report; initial

92225-50 Ophthalmoscopy [for second eye]

See the next bullet point for the appropriate use of modifier 50 under Medicare guidelines.

- Medicare guidelines for the use of modifier 50 differ from many third-party payers' accepted protocol. In part, the new definition of modifier 50 found in the 1999 CPT code book reflects the Medicare perspective in the modifier's use for Medicare claims, and other major third-party payers may begin to follow suit. The *Medicare Carriers Manual*, CAR3 4827.B states, "If a procedure is not identified by its terminology as a bilateral procedure (or unilateral or bilateral), report the procedure with modifier 50. Report such procedures as a single line item." For instance, if the bilateral ophthalmoscopy procedures cited in the previous bullet were performed on a Medicare patient, both procedures would be reported as follows:

92225-50 Ophthalmoscopy, extended, with retinal drawing (e.g., for retinal detachment, melanoma), with interpretation and report; initial

The second, or bilateral, procedure is inherent in the one-line item by the 50 modifier being appended to the appropriate procedure code.

Note: Some Medicare carriers will also accept bilateral procedures reported as two-line items with the right (RT) and left (LT) HCPCS Level II modifiers appended to the respective procedure codes.

- CPT codes for use with modifier 50, unless limited by the payer, are 10021–69990, 70010–79999, and 90281–99600, if appropriate.

51 MULTIPLE PROCEDURES

When multiple procedures, other than evaluation and management services, are performed at the same session by the same provider, the primary procedure or service may be reported as listed. The additional procedure(s) or service(s) may be identified by appending the modifier 51 to the additional procedure or service code(s).

Using the Modifier Correctly

- Modifier 51 is used to indicate that more than one surgical service or procedure was performed by the same physician on the same patient on the same date of service.
- Multiple surgeries are separate procedures performed by the same physician on the same day or operative session. A multiple surgical payment reduction is applied by Medicare as the major surgery includes payment for patient preparation time and services. Report the major procedure without the 51 modifier and additional procedures with the 51 modifier. Medicare determines the major

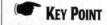

KEY POINT

The following medical procedure codes are considered add-on procedures by most third-party payers. These codes generally cannot be reported in isolation of a primary procedure. As the information under coding tips explains, the modifier 51 is not reportable with add-on codes. The following codes can be found in the 2004 CPT manual in appendix E, "Summary of CPT Add-on Codes." Codes listed in appendix E of the CPT manual are also identified throughout the CPT manual by the + symbol.

90472	90474	90781	92547
92608	92973	92974	92978
92979	92981	92984	92996
92998	93320	93321	93325
93571	93572	93609	93613
93621	93622	93623	93662
95920	95962	95967	95973
96412	96423	96570	95975
96571	97546	99100	99116
99135	99140	99290	99292
99354	99355	99356	99357
99358	99359	99602	

procedure based upon the highest Medicare fee schedule amount of the surgeries performed/reported. The major procedure is paid based on 100 percent of the fee schedule amount. Payment for the additional procedures are based on 50 percent of the Medicare fee schedule amount. Some surgical procedures are not subject to multiple surgery reduction guidelines.

- Modifier 51 applies only to certain codes.
- Because of the nature of the CPT code book definition for EEG testing, multiple component tests are defined. When performed at the same session, use the 51 modifier, indicating that multiple procedures were performed at the same session.
- Pulmonary stress testing (CPT code 94621) is a comprehensive stress test with a number of component tests separately defined in the CPT manual. It is inappropriate to separately code EKG monitoring, spirometric parameters performed before, during and after exercise, CO_2 production, etc., when performed as part of a progressive pulmonary exercise test. It is also inappropriate to bill for a cardiac stress test and the component codes used to perform a routine pulmonary stress test when a comprehensive pulmonary stress test was performed. If using a standard exercise protocol, serial electro-cardiograms are obtained, and a separate report describing a cardiac stress test (i.e., a professional component) is included in the medical record, both a cardiac and pulmonary stress test could be billed. Modifier 51 is appended with the second procedure if both tests are billed. Both tests must satisfy the requirement for medical necessity.

Incorrect Use of the Modifier

- Using modifier 51 on procedures that are considered components or incidental to a primary procedure. The intraoperative services, incidental surgeries or components of more major surgeries are not separately billable.
- Using modifier 51 in instances in which two or more physicians each performs distinctly different, unrelated surgeries on the same day/same patient (e.g., multiple trauma cases). Modifier 51 is used only if one of the surgeons individually performs multiple surgeries.
- Using modifier 51 with CPT codes 93539–93556. These procedures describe injection procedures during cardiac catheterization and imaging supervision and interpretation and are considered modifier 51 exempt when reported.

Coding Tips

- When multiple procedures, other than E/M services, are performed on the same day or at the same session by the same provider, report the primary procedure or service. Modifier 51 is appended to the appropriate CPT code for the additional service(s) or procedure(s).
- Modifier 51 should not be used with add-on codes. Add-on codes are procedures performed in addition to the main procedure. These codes represent procedures that cannot be performed alone. Examples of words to look for as clues to add-on procedures are each additional, list in addition to, and second lesion.
- CPT codes for use with modifier 51, unless limited by the payer are 00100–01999, 10021–69990, 70010–79999, and 90281–99600, when appropriate.

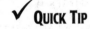

QUICK TIP

Hospital ASC and Outpatient Coders

Modifier 51 is not applicable in hospital ASC or hospital outpatient facilities in accordance with CPT's modifiers approved for ASC outpatient hospital use.

52 REDUCED SERVICES

Under certain circumstances a service or procedure is partially reduced or eliminated at the physician's discretion. Under these circumstances the service provided can be identified by its usual procedure number and the addition of the modifier 52, signifying that the service is reduced. This provides a means of reporting reduced services without disturbing the identification of the basic service. **Note:** For hospital outpatient reporting of a previously scheduled procedure/service that is partially reduced or canceled as a result of extenuating circumstances or those that threaten the well-being of the patient prior to or after administration of anesthesia, see modifiers 73 and 74.

Using the Modifier Correctly

- Modifier is used for reporting services that were partially reduced or eliminated at the physician's election. Documentation should be present in the medical record explaining the reduction.
- Modifier 52 is used to indicate that a procedure or service was performed at a lesser level. A concise statement that describes how the service differs from the normal procedure must be included with the claim.
- Procedure code 93922 describes a bilateral procedure. However, sometimes the procedure cannot be performed as described in the CPT code book. For example, if a noninvasive physiologic study is performed on a patient who previously had an above the knee amputation, append the modifier 52 to code 93922 to indicate that this test was not performed in its entirety.
- Provocative testing (CPT code 91052) can be expedited during GI endoscopy. When this is performed, append modifier 52 to CPT code 91052 indicating that a reduced level of service was performed.

Incorrect Use of the Modifier

- Using modifier 52 for terminated procedures. This modifier is intended for procedures that accomplished some result, but less than expected for the procedure.
- Using modifier 52 on an E/M code for certain third-party payer claims. Many insurance companies do not recognize modifier 52 on this type of service. Check with individual payers for the accepted use of modifier 52 on an E/M code.
- Using modifier 52 on a time-based code (i.e., critical care, psychotherapy, anesthesia), automated organ or disease panels or codes that specifically states "limited" (e.g., duplex sonography). Check with carriers to see if they recognize modifier 52 with these codes and find out their policy for its use. In some cases, there are alternative choices for coding a lesser service, so modifier 52 would not be reported.

Coding Tips

- Modifier 52 is used to indicate under certain circumstances, a service or procedure is partially reduced or eliminated at the physician's discretion.
- The use of this modifier may affect payment. For exams considered global, this modifier is informational only and does not affect payment. For other situations, such as aborted procedures, a reduction in payment may occur.
- The 52 modifier is used for a reduced service and is not a modifier to be used just because the fee is reduced to a patient due to inability to pay.

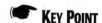

KEY POINT

The *Medicare Carriers Manual* (See CMS Web-based manual, pub 100) states, in part, that when procedures for which services performed are significantly less than usually required, [these services] may be billed with modifier 52 ... [and] procedures reported with this modifier should include the following documentation:

- A concise statement about how the service or procedure differs from the usual
- The operative report

Claims reported with modifier 52 that do not include the required documentation will be processed as if there were no modifiers reported.

QUICK TIP

Hospital ASC and Outpatient Coders
Per Medicare, modifier 52, Reduced service, is used in the hospital outpatient department to identify a procedure not requiring anesthesia (meaning general, regional, or local) that was terminated after the patient was prepared for the procedure (including any sedation). Reimbursement for modifier 52 procedures is 50 percent.

- CPT codes for use with modifier 52 (unless limited by the payer) are 99201–99499 (except for Medicare), 10021–69990, 70010–79999, 80048–89399, and 90281–99600 (except psychotherapy), when appropriate.

53   Discontinued Procedure

Under certain circumstances, the physician may elect to terminate a surgical or diagnostic procedure. Due to extenuating circumstances or those that threaten the well-being of the patient, it may be necessary to indicate that a surgical or diagnostic procedure was started but discontinued. This circumstance may be reported by adding modifier 53 to the code reported by the physician for the discontinued procedure. **Note:** This modifier is not used to report the elective cancellation of a procedure prior to the patient's anesthesia induction and/or surgical preparation in the operating suite. For outpatient hospital/ASC reporting of a previously scheduled procedure/service that is partially reduced or cancelled as a result of extenuating circumstances or those that threaten the well-being of the patient prior to or after administration of anesthesia, see modifiers 73 and 74.

Using the Modifier Correctly
- Modifier 53 is used when a procedure was actually started but had to be discontinued before completion. For example, a cardiac catheterization might be discontinued when the catheter could not be advanced into the heart and was withdrawn without obtaining any diagnostic data. The claim should be accompanied by the operative/procedure report so that a determination of the work involved can be made for pricing purposes.
- If the procedure was discontinued after anesthesia was induced, report the aborted procedure using the appropriate CPT code with modifier 53.
- If a surgery is discontinued due to uncontrollable bleeding, hypotension, or neurologic impairment—situations that threaten the well-being of the patient—append modifier 53 to the surgical procedure code.
- Modifier 53 applies to the physician's office as well. All procedures billed with the 53 modifier may require documentation to be submitted with the claim.

Incorrect Use of the Modifier
- Using modifier 53 to report the elective cancellation of a procedure prior to the patient's anesthesia induction and/or surgical preparation in the operative suite.
- Using modifier 53 when a procedure is prematurely terminated prior to the induction of anesthesia. The correct modifier to report these services is modifier 52.
- Using modifier 53 on an E/M code. Many insurance companies do not recognize the modifier 53 on this type of service. Check with individual payers for use of modifier 53 on an E/M code.
- Using modifier 53 on a time-based code (i.e., critical care, psychotherapy, anesthesia), automated organ or disease panels or codes that specifically state "limited" (e.g., duplex sonography). Check with the carriers to see if they recognize modifier 53 in these scenarios, and find out their policy for its use. In some cases, there are alternative choices for coding a lesser service, so modifier 53 would not be appended.

Quick Tip

Hospital and Outpatient Coders
Modifier 53 is not applicable in hospital ASC or hospital outpatient facilities in accordance with CPT modifiers approved for ASC outpatient hospital use.

Coding Tips

- Modifier 53 is used when under extenuating circumstances or those that threaten the well-being of the patient, the physician may elect to terminate a diagnostic or medical procedure. Use this modifier when it may be necessary to indicate that a diagnostic or medical procedure was started but was discontinued.
- For aborted or discontinued procedures, the appropriate ICD-9-CM diagnosis code (V64.1, V64.2, or V64.3) is reported. Follow individual third-party payer guidelines, as some payers and managed care organizations do not accept V codes.
- CPT codes for use with modifier 53 are 00100–01999, 10021–69990, 70010–79999, 80048–89399, and 90281–99600 unless limited by the payer.

Clinical Example

A patient presented for day surgery for an endomyocardial biopsy for his yearly follow up exam for a heart transplant he had five years ago. The patient was prepped and the procedure started without difficulty. The physician threaded the catheter to the heart through a central IV line inserted in the femoral vein. The physician was about to take samples when the patient exhibited a ventricular arrhythmia on EKG monitor. The surgeon terminated the procedure due to high risk to the patient. The patient will be admitted for observation and treatment.

CPT code 93505-53 is submitted.

55 POSTOPERATIVE MANAGEMENT ONLY

When one physician performs the postoperative management and another physician has performed the surgical procedure, the postoperative component may be identified by adding the modifier 55 to the usual procedure number.

Using the Modifier Correctly

- Use with procedure codes to indicate that only the postoperative care was performed (i.e., another physician performed the procedure). In this case, the postoperative component may be identified by adding the modifier 55 to the CPT procedure code.
- Modifier 55 is appended if a physician does not perform the procedure but does provide a portion of the postoperative care. List the assumed date in item 19 of the CMS-1500 claim form, the procedure code with the 55 modifier in item 24d, the date of service in the from and to fields of 24a and one unit of service in item 24g. Electronic billing software should have a narrative data field for this date in the HAO record. Information from item 19 must be included so the payer will know the date the physician assumed care.
- Use modifier 55 after discharge of the patient from the hospital if applicable, and only after the patient has been seen in follow-up.
- Providers need not state on the claim that care has been transferred. However, the *Medicare Carriers Manual*, CAR3, section 4822.B, See CMS Web-based manual, pub 100-4, chapter 12, sections, 40.4 and 40.5) states the date in which care was relinquished or assumed, as applicable, must be shown on the claim.

Hospital ASC and Outpatient Coders
Modifiers 54 and 55 are not applicable in hospital ASC or hospital outpatient facilities in accordance with CPT modifiers approved for ASC outpatient hospital use.

When one physician performs a patient's surgical service and another provides the postoperative management, an agreement for the transfer of care must be retained in the Medicare beneficiary's medical records. This agreement can be in the form of a letter, discharge summary, chart notation or other written documentation, but in any case, both providers must retain a copy of the agreement.

- Where a transfer of postoperative care occurs, the receiving physician cannot bill for any part of the global services until he or she has provided at least one service. Once the physician sees the patient, that physician may bill using the 55 modifier for the period beginning with the date on which he or she assumes care of the patient.
- For each surgical CPT code, third-party payers have established a certain percentage for each of the three components (i.e., preoperative, intraoperative, and postoperative). If the split care modifiers (54, 55, and 56) are used, these percentages help determine payment.

Incorrect Use of the Modifier

- Using modifier 55 on the procedure code if a physician other than the performing physician provides the inpatient postoperative care when the transfer of care occurs immediately after the procedure. The physician other than the performing physician should bill these inpatient services using the subsequent hospital care codes (99231–99233).

Coding Tips

- At times, more than one physician will provide the services that are included in the global surgical package. This may occur when one physician performs the surgical or medical procedure and a second physician provides the follow-up care. The 55 modifier is added to the procedure code if one physician does the procedure but another physician provides the postoperative care.
- The 55 modifier is an indicator that multiple physicians are involved in the patient's procedural care. Each physician must report the service he or she provided so that the correct payments will be made for each claim upon submission. For example, Medicare payment is limited to the same total amount as would have been paid if one physician provided all the care, regardless of the number of caregivers. Payment for modifier 55 will be limited to the amount allowed for postoperative services only. In addition, when more than one physician is providing postoperative care, each physician would be paid based on the number of postoperative days that each cared for the patient (e.g., using a 90-day postoperative period, a 45- to 45-day split, 30- to 60-day split, 10- to 60- to 20-day split, etc.).
- The 55 modifier is appended to the procedure code only after the first postoperative visit is provided by the physician performing the postoperative management.
- CPT codes for use with modifier 55 are appropriate codes in the surgery section (10040–69990) and in the medicine section (90281–99600), unless limited by the third-party payer.

Clinical Examples

Example #1:

A cardiothoracic surgeon performed a percutaneous balloon valvuloplasty on the patient's pulmonary valve due to pulmonary valve insufficiency. The surgeon followed this patient in the hospital but upon discharge wrote a transfer of care order to another physician who will follow up with postoperative care.

The physician who acquires this patient for postoperative care would report CPT code 92990-55 after the first postdischarge visit with this patient.

> ✓ **QUICK TIP**
>
> Under federal guidelines, when a patient's surgical service and the subsequent postoperative care are rendered in different Medicare carrier localities, each service must be billed to the respective carrier servicing the different payment localities. Both modifier 54 and modifier 55 are appropriate for this kind of service reporting. For example, if a surgery is performed in carrier A's region but the postoperative management is provided in carrier B's locality, the surgery would be billed to carrier A with modifier 54 appended to the applicable CPT procedure codes, and the postoperative care would be billed to carrier B by reporting modifier 55 with the applicable CPT procedure codes. This guideline must be followed whether the services are performed by the same physician or physician group, or whether the services are performed by different physicians or physician groups.

> ✓ **QUICK TIP**
>
> Since the Medicare fee schedule amount for surgical procedures includes all component services that comprise the global surgical package (pre-, intra-, and postoperative services), the sum of the Medicare approved amount for all of the physicians involved in the patient's care, even when fragmented into these components, will not exceed the typical global amount allowed if only one physician were to provide the entire surgical package. An exception to this policy occurs when the surgeon performs only the surgery and another physician—other than the surgeon—provides both the preoperative and postoperative inpatient care. This can result in a total payment to all involved physicians that is higher than the global surgery allowed amount.

Example #2:
An atrial septectomy, transvenous method, balloon (Rashkind type) and a cardiac catheterization were performed for a patient's congenital atrial septal defect. The surgeon will transfer postoperative care to a cardiologist once the patient is discharged from the hospital.

The cardiologist would report CPT code 92992-55 after the first post discharge visit with this patient.

56   PREOPERATIVE MANAGEMENT ONLY

When one physician performs the preoperative care and evaluation and another physician performs the surgical procedure, the preoperative component may be identified by adding the modifier 56 to the usual procedure number.

Using the Modifier Correctly
- The modifier 56 is used to the usual procedure code when one physician performs the preoperative care and evaluation and another physician performs the surgical or medical procedure.
- For each surgical CPT code, third-party payers have established a certain percentage for each of the three components (i.e., preoperative, intraoperative, and postoperative). If the split care modifiers (54, 55, and 56) are used, these percentages help determine appropriate payment.
- Medicare carriers and other third-party payers should be consulted for their instructions on the appropriate use of this modifier. Payment for this modifier is included in the Medicare allowable for the surgery. If a different physician performs the preoperative service, use the appropriate E/M code. Follow your carrier's instructions on the use of this modifier.

Incorrect Use of the Modifier
- Using modifier 56 with an E/M service code.

Coding Tips
- At times, more than one physician will provide the services that are included in the global surgical package. This may occur when one physician performs the surgical or medical procedure and a second physician provides the follow-up care. Modifier 56 is applied to the code used for the surgery or the procedure if the physician provides only preoperative service.
- Modifier 56 is rarely used for services found in the medicine section of the CPT code book, and it should only be used on procedures with global periods.
- CPT codes for use with modifier 56 are only 10021–69990 unless the third-party payer also accepts the modifier on medical services.

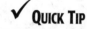

Hospital ASC and Outpatient Coders
Modifier 56 is not applicable in hospital ASC or hospital outpatient facilities in accordance with CPT modifiers approved for ASC outpatient hospital use.

57   DECISION FOR SURGERY

An evaluation and management service that resulted in the initial decision to perform the surgery may be identified by adding the modifier 57 to the appropriate level of E/M service.

Using the Modifier Correctly
- Modifier 57 is added to the appropriate level of E/M service or opthalmological service that resulted in the initial decision to perform the surgery or procedure.

- For Medicare claims, modifier 57 should be used only in cases in which the decision for surgery was made during the preoperative period of a surgical procedure with a 90-day postoperative period (i.e., major surgery). The preoperative period is defined as the day before and the day of the procedure.

Incorrect Use of the Modifier
- Appending modifier 57 to a surgical procedure code. It is only to be reported with E/M and specific opthalmological service codes.
- Because of Medicare's requirements, this modifier is often misused by placing it on an E/M service performed on the same day as a minor procedure. Do not use modifier 57 on the E/M visit furnished during the preoperative period of a minor procedure (defined by Medicare as having a zero- to 10-day postoperative period). According to Medicare rules, where the decision to perform the minor procedure is typically done immediately before the service, it is considered a routine preoperative service and a visit or consultation is not billed in addition to the procedure.
- Attaching modifier 57 to the hospital visit code for the day before surgery or day of surgery when the decision to perform the major surgical procedure (as defined by Medicare) was made in advance of the surgery.

Coding Tips
- Modifier 57 is not a surgical modifier; append this modifier only to E/M and opthalmological service codes 92012 and 92014.
- A clear understanding of the payers' rules is necessary in order to assign this modifier correctly. The CPT code book simply defines 57 as a modifier to represent an E/M service that resulted in the initial decision to perform surgery. Medicare states it should be used to indicate that the E/M service performed the day before or the day of surgery resulted in the decision for major surgery (i.e., those with a 90-day follow-up period). Medicare guidelines instruct coders to use modifier 25 if the decision for surgery is made on the same day as a minor surgery or procedure (i.e., in those with a zero- to 10-day follow-up period).
- This modifier is one of a group of CPT modifiers (24, 25, 57, 58, 78, and 79) that serve to identify an E/M service or procedure furnished during a global surgical period that is normally not a part of the global surgery package.
- CPT codes for use with the modifier 57 are 92002–92014, and 99201–99499 unless limited by the payer, if appropriate.

58   STAGED OR RELATED PROCEDURE OR SERVICE BY THE SAME PHYSICIAN DURING THE POSTOPERATIVE PERIOD

The physician may need to indicate that the performance of a procedure or service during the postoperative period was: a) planned prospectively at the time of the original procedure (staged); b) more extensive than the original procedure; or c) for therapy following a diagnostic surgical procedure. This circumstance may be reported by adding the modifier 58 to the staged or related procedure. **Note:** This modifier is not used to report the treatment of a problem that requires a return to the operating room. See modifier 78.

Using the Modifier Correctly
- Modifier 58 is used only when the second or related services are performed during the postoperative period of the original procedure.

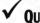

Hospital ASC and Outpatient Coders
Facilities should use 25 in place of modifier 57 for the emergency department visit on the same day as a procedure that has a status of indicator of S or T. Modifier 57 is not a valid hospital/ASC modifier.

Use modifier 58 only when the subsequent procedure occurs within the postoperative global surgery period.

Modifier 58 must be used for purposes of distinguishing procedures performed by the original surgeon or provider during the postoperative period of the original (first) procedure, within the constraints of the modifier's definition. These procedures cannot be repeat operations (unless the procedures are more extensive than the original procedure) and cannot be for the treatment of complications requiring a return trip to the operating room.

- Modifier 58 is for use in a global period of another procedure. It would be used very rarely with the medicine codes. The staged procedure would have to be:
  —planned prospectively at the time of the original procedure
  —more extensive than the original procedure
  —for therapy following a diagnostic surgical procedure
- A new postoperative period begins when the next procedure in the staged procedure series is billed.
- If more than one physician is involved in a staged procedure, each physician must submit the claim using the modifiers 58 and 52 (reduced service). These claims are subject to individual consideration and payment calculation is based on the percentage of the procedure each physician performs.

Incorrect Use of the Modifier
- Using modifier 58 to report the treatment of a problem that requires a return to the operating room. See modifier 78 for this purpose.
- Using modifier 58 for unrelated procedures performed during the postoperative period of the original (first) procedure or service. See modifier 79 for unrelated procedures performed by the same physician during the postoperative period, or modifiers 51 and 59, as appropriate, for multiple procedures and distinct procedural service for procedures performed by another physician during the postoperative period of the original surgery. (**Note:** For repeat procedures performed by another physician, see modifier 77.)

Coding Tips
- To report a staged or related procedure add the modifier 58. Failure to use this modifier when appropriate may result in denial of the subsequent surgery or procedure claim.
- Do not use modifier 58 with CPT procedure codes that are described as one or more services. These procedures in the CPT code book are considered multiple sessions or are otherwise defined as including multiple services or event. The Medicare fee schedule RVU was established based on the total procedure. Therefore, separate reimbursement may not be made for each segment of the procedure even if it is for one or more services.
- CPT codes for use with modifier 58 are 10021–69990, 70010–79999, and 90281–99600 unless limited by the payer.

QUICK TIP

Modifier 58, among others, was the recent target of an investigation by various Medicare carriers across the country (under the direction of CMS). Errors in reporting modifier 58 occurred most often by general surgeons, ophthalmologists, and orthopaedic surgeons, who were found to be misusing the modifier to bill for postoperative complications treated in the physician office setting. Unless the complications require a return trip to the operating room, these services are included in the global surgical package by Medicare.

59   DISTINCT PROCEDURAL SERVICE

Under certain circumstances, the physician may need to indicate that a procedure or service was distinct or independent from other services performed on the same day. Modifier 59 is used to identify procedures/services that are not normally reported together, but are appropriate under the circumstances. This may represent a different session or patient encounter, different procedure or surgery, different site or organ system, separate incision/excision, separate lesion, or separate injury (or area of injury in extensive injuries) not ordinarily encountered or performed on the same day by the same physician. However, when another already established modifier is appropriate it should be used rather than modifier 59. Only if no more descriptive modifier is available, and the use of modifier 59 best explains the circumstances, should modifier 59 be used.

Ingenix Coding Lab: Understanding Modifiers

KEY POINT

Use modifier 59 only when the subsequent procedure occurs on the same date as another procedure by the same provider.

KEY POINT

Modifier 59 was established (and replaced the HCPCS Level II temporary modifier GB) to demonstrate that multiple yet distinct services were provided to a patient on the same date of service by the same provider. Because distinct procedures or services rendered on the same day by the same physician cannot be easily identified and therefore properly adjudicated by simply listing the CPT procedure codes, modifier 59 assists the third-party payer or Medicare carrier in applying the appropriate reimbursement protocol. If the modifier is not used in these circumstances, a denial of services may ensue, with the explanation of benefits stating, for instance for Medicare claims, "Medicare does not pay for this service because it is part of another service that was performed at the same time."

Using the Modifier Correctly

- Modifier 59 is used when a billing a combination of codes that would normally not be billed together. This modifier indicates that the ordinarily bundled code represents a service done at a different anatomic site or at a different session on the same date. This may represent:
  —different session or patient encounter
  —different procedure or service/same day
  —different site or organ system (e.g., a skin graft and an allograft in different locations)
  —separate incision/excision
  —separate lesion (e.g., a biopsy of skin on the neck is performed at the same session as an excision of a 1.0 cm benign lesion of the face)
  —separate injury

- Modifier 59 is used only on the procedure that is designated as the distinct procedural service. The physician needs to document that a procedure or service was distinct or separate from other services performed on the same day.

- The documentation must be clear as to the separate and distinct procedure before appending modifier 59 to a code. This modifier allows the code to bypass edits; therefore, appropriate documentation must be present in the record. **Note:** Medicare uses CCI screens when editing claims for possible unbundling. Under the CCI edits, specific codes have been identified that should not be billed together.

- Modifier 59 is used only if another modifier does not describe the situation more accurately.

- In the case of chemotherapy administration, fluids such as saline or dextrose solutions may be necessary to maintain line patency or flush lines between different agents given at the same session. Do not separately bill for infusion of these fluids. However, if fluid administration is medically necessary for therapeutic reasons (e.g., hydration or preservation of renal function) and provided sequentially, not concurrently with the course of a transfusion or chemotherapy, report this service and append the code separately with the 59 modifier.

- A number of therapeutic and diagnostic cardiovascular procedures (e.g., CPT codes 92950–92998, 93501–93545, 93600–93624, and 93640–93652) routinely utilize intravenous or intraarterial vascular access, routinely require electrocardiographic monitoring and frequently require agents administered by injection or infusion techniques. Accordingly, do not bill separately these services for routine access, monitoring, injection or infusion. Fluoroscopic guidance procedures are routinely used during invasive intravascular procedures and also are included in those services. In unique circumstances, where these services are performed and are not an integral part of the procedure, report the appropriate code with the 59 modifier. When supervision and interpretation codes are identified in the CPT code book for a given procedure, bill these separately.

- Polysomnography requires at least one central and usually several EEG electrodes. EEG procurement for polysomnography (sleep staging) differs greatly from that required for diagnostic EEG testing (i.e., speed of paper, number of channels, etc.). Accordingly, do not bill EEG testing with polysomnography unless performed separately. Bill the EEG tests, if rendered, with a separate report with the 59 modifier, indicating that this represents a different session from the sleep study.

©2003 Ingenix, Inc.
CPT only ©2003 American Medical Association. All Rights Reserved.

- Biofeedback services involve the use of electromyographic techniques to detect and record muscle activity. The CPT codes 95860–95872 (EMG) are not billed with biofeedback services based on the use of electromyography during a biofeedback session. If an EMG is performed as a separate medically necessary service for the diagnosis or follow-up of organic muscle dysfunction, bill the appropriate EMG codes (e.g., CPT codes 95860–95872). The 59 modifier is appended to indicate that the service performed was a separately identifiable diagnostic service. Reporting only an objective electromyographic response to biofeedback is not sufficient to bill the codes referable to EMG.

Incorrect Use of the Modifier
- Using modifier 59 with E/M codes.
- Using modifier 59 as a replacement for modifiers 24, 25, 78, or 79.
- Using modifier 59 when another modifier best describes the distinct service.

Coding Tips
- Modifier 59 is used to indicate that a procedure or service was distinct or independent from other services performed on the same day.
- If there is not a more descriptive modifier available, and the use of modifier 59 best explains the circumstance, then append modifier 59.
- When a procedure or service that is designated as a separate procedure in the CPT code book is carried out independently or considered to be unrelated or distinct from the other services provided at the same session, it may be reported by appending the 59 modifier to the separate procedure code to indicate that the procedure is not considered to be a component of another procedure, but instead is a distinct, independent procedure.
- CPT codes for use with 59 modifier are 00100–01999, 10021–69990, 70010–79999, 80048–89399, and 90281–99600, when appropriate. unless limited by the payer.

Clinical Example
A patient presents who is being treated for colon cancer with chemotherapy. Due to the patient's type of cancer and the various routes of administering the agents, attach the -59 modifier to the lesser valued technique indicating that separate agents were administered by different techniques (96408–96450).

76 Repeat Procedure by Same Physician

The physician may need to indicate that a procedure or service was repeated subsequent to the original procedure or service. This circumstance may be reported by adding the modifier 76 to the repeated procedure/service.

Using the Modifier Correctly
- Modifier 76 is appended to a code when the same physician repeats the same service, usually on the same day. This modifier can be used whenever the circumstances warrant this information.
- This modifier is used to indicate that a repeat procedure was necessary and that does not represent a duplicate bill.
- Medicare does not recognize procedure codes 92525 (evaluation of swallowing and oral function for feeding) and 92526 (treatment of swallowing dysfunction and/or oral function for feeding) as repeat procedures. Therefore, do not report modifier 76 in conjunction with these services.

Hospital ASC and Outpatient Coders

Medicare's instructions for modifiers 76 and 77 in hospital ASC or hospital outpatient facilities include in the definition procedures "repeated in a separate operative session on the same calendar day." Use modifier 76 for same physician/same day and modifier 77 for another physician/same day. The procedure must be the same procedure.

Modifier 76, among others, was the recent target of an investigation by various Medicare carriers across the country (under the direction of CMS). Errors in reporting modifier 76 occurred most often during this investigation by cardiologists, who showed a trend of misusing the modifier to bill for cardiac catheterization codes 93555 and 93556.

KEY POINT

When determining the extent of a global surgical period for major surgeries and procedures (i.e., those with a 90-day follow-up period), use the following guidelines set forth by the *Medicare Carriers Manual*. (See CMS Web-based manual, pub 100). These guidelines are likewise followed by many state Medicaid programs and other major third-party payers. First, count one day immediately prior to the day of the major surgery. Then, count the day the surgical procedure is carried out, and finally count the 90 days immediately following the day of surgery. For example:

Date of surgery: April 24, 2001

Preoperative period: April 23, 2001

Last day of postoperative period: July 23, 2001

When determining the extent of a global surgical period for minor surgeries and procedures (i.e., those with zero- to 10-day follow-up periods), use the following guidelines set forth by the *Medicare Carriers Manual* (See CMS Web-based manual, pub 100). These guidelines, as well as the above-stated major surgery/procedure guidelines, are recognized by many state Medicaid programs and other major third-party payers. First, count the day the minor procedure is carried out, and then count the appropriate number of days following the date of the procedure. For example:

Date of surgery (for a procedure with a 10-day postoperative period): April 24, 2001

Last day of postoperative period: May 4, 2001.

✓ QUICK TIP

Hospital ASC and Outpatient Coders
Medicare's instructions for modifiers 76 and 77 in hospital ASC or hospital outpatient facilities include in the definition procedures "repeated in a separate operative session on the same calendar day." Use modifier 76 for same physician/same day and modifier 77 for another physician/same day. The procedure must be the same procedure.

Incorrect Use of the Modifier
- Using modifier 76 to indicate repositioning or replacement 14 days after the initial insertion or replacement of an existing pacemaker or defibrillator. Modifier 76 is not reported with pacemaker or defibrillator codes after 14 days as these are considered new, not repeat, services.

Coding Tips
- Modifier 76 is added to the repeat service to indicate that a procedure or service was repeated subsequent to the original service. An explanation of the medical necessity for the repeat procedure is necessary.
- For Medicare clinical laboratory tests, same day, see modifier 91 in the pathology and laboratory chapter.
- CPT codes for use with modifier 76 are 10021–69990, 70010–79999, and 90281–99600, when appropriate unless limited by the payer.

77   REPEAT PROCEDURE BY ANOTHER PHYSICIAN

The physician may need to indicate that a basic procedure or service performed by another physician had to be repeated. This situation may be reported by adding modifier 77 to the repeated procedure/service.

Using the Modifier Correctly
- Modifier 77 is appended to a CPT code when the same service (same CPT code) that was already performed by another physician is repeated by a different physician; usually on the same date of service. This modifier can be used whenever the circumstances warrant this information.

Incorrect Use of the Modifier
- Using modifier 77 to indicate repositioning or replacement 14 days after the initial insertion or replacement of an existing pacemaker or defibrillator. Modifier 77 is not reported with pacemaker or defibrillator codes after 14 days because these are considered new, not repeat services.

Coding Tips
- Modifier 77 is added to the repeated service to indicate that a procedure performed by another physician needed to be repeated by a second physician. An explanation of the medical necessity for the repeat service is necessary.
- Modifier 77 does not guarantee reimbursement of the repeated services as other third-party payer regulations (such as medical necessity) are still applicable.
- CPT codes for use with modifier 77 are 10021–69990, 70010–79999, and 90281–99600, when appropriate unless limited by the payer.

78   RETURN TO OPERATING ROOM FOR A RELATED PROCEDURE DURING THE POSTOPERATIVE PERIOD

The physician may need to indicate that another procedure was performed during the postoperative period of the initial procedure. When this subsequent procedure is related to the first, and requires the use of the operating room, it may be reported by adding the modifier 78 to the related procedure. (For repeat procedures on the same day, see modifier 76.)

Using the Modifier Correctly
- Using modifier 78 when treatment for complications requires a return trip to the operating room. Use the CPT code that best describes the procedure performed during the return trip. If no such code exists, the unspecified procedure code in the correct series should be used (e.g., 47999, 67999, etc.).
- Modifier 78 is used on procedure codes to indicate that another procedure was performed during the postoperative period of the initial procedure, was related to the first and required the use of the operating room.
- If the patient is returned to the operating room after the initial operative session, even if on the same day as the original surgery, for one or more additional procedures as a result of complications from the original surgery, use the 78 modifier.

Incorrect Use of the Modifier
- Using modifier 78 on the procedure code when the original surgery is reported. If the identical procedure was repeated, modifier 76 is used.
- Only using modifier 78 for complications of surgery. The CPT code book definition for this modifier does not limit its use to treatment for complications.
- Using this modifier to bill Medicare for a procedure not performed in the operating room (unless the patient's condition was so critical there would be insufficient time for transportation to an operating room).

Coding Tips
- Modifier 78 is added to the procedure code when the subsequent procedure is related to the first and requires the use of an operating room. Failure to use this modifier when appropriate may result in denial of the subsequent procedure.
- If a CPT code exists for the related procedure, modifier 78 is appended to it. If no CPT code exists for the related procedure, append the modifier to an unlisted procedure code. For Medicare patients, payment is limited to the amount allowed for intraoperative services only. **Note:** For each surgical CPT code, most third-party payers have established a certain reimbursement percentage for each of the three components (i.e., preoperative, intraoperative and postoperative).
- Do not use modifier 78 if treatment for postoperative complications did not require a return trip to the operating room.
- A new postoperative period does not begin with the use of the 78 modifier.
- An operating room is defined by CMS as a place of service specifically equipped and staffed for the sole purpose of performing procedures. This includes cardiac catheterization suites, laser suites, and endoscopy suites. It does not include a patient's room, a minor treatment room, a recovery room or an ICU.
- CPT codes for use with the modifier 78 are 10021–69990, 70010–79999, and 90281–99600, when appropriate.

Clinical Example
A patient is two days postsurgery for percutaneous balloon valvuloplasty of the aortic valve (92986) and suddenly experienced severe chest pain and shortness of breath. The surgeon was notified and arrived within 20 minutes. The patient was returned to the operating room where a pulmonary artery embolectomy with cardiopulmonary bypass was performed.

CPT code 33910-78 is submitted for the surgery resulting from complications related to the original procedure. This modifier will affect reimbursement. For Medicare and

Hospital ASC and Outpatient Coders
Medicare's instructions for modifiers 78 and 79 in hospital ASC or hospital outpatient facilities include in the definition procedures "return to the operating room on the same day." Use modifier 78 for a procedure related to the initial procedure on the same day and modifier 79 for a procedure on the same day that is unrelated to the initial procedure.

Modifier 78, among others, was the recent target of an investigation by various Medicare carriers across the country (under the direction of CMS). Errors in reporting modifier 78 occurred most often by ophthalmologists, who were found to be misusing the modifier to bill for postoperative complications treated in the physician office setting. Unless the complications require a return trip to the operating room, these services are included in the global surgical package by Medicare.

Ingenix Coding Lab: Understanding Modifiers

major third-party payers, the surgeon will only receive the intraoperative percentage of the total allowable for the procedure code. The global period will not change from the original procedure.

79   Unrelated Procedure or Service by the Same Physician During the Postoperative Period

The physician may need to indicate that the performance of a procedure or service during the postoperative period was unrelated to the original procedure. This circumstance may be reported by using the modifier 79. (For repeat procedures on the same day, see modifier 76.)

Using the Modifier Correctly
- Use the modifier 79 on procedure codes only to indicate that an unrelated procedure was performed by the same physician during a postoperative period of the original procedure.

Incorrect Use of the Modifier
- Using the modifier 79 to describe a related procedure performed in a postoperative period by the same surgeon.

Coding Tips
- Use modifier 79 to indicate that the procedure performed by the physician is unrelated to the original service or procedure. A different diagnosis code should be reported, linked to the unrelated procedure. Failure to use this modifier when appropriate may result in denial of the subsequent surgery or procedure claim.
- It is important that each line item include the necessary modifier when appropriate. For example, if the physician has performed two unrelated surgical procedures that fall in the postoperative period of another surgery the physician performed, apply the 79 modifier to both surgery codes, not just the first.
- CPT codes for use with the modifier 79 are 10021–69990, 70010–79999, and 90281–99600 if appropriate and unless limited by the payer.

Clinical Example
The patient was in the postoperative period for a Park septostomy (CPT code 92993). The surgeon performed a flexible fiberoptic laryngoscopy for removal of a lesion on day 40 of the postoperative period.

Submit CPT code 31578-79. This procedure was not related to the original procedure. The use of the 79 modifier will start a new global period. Reimbursement should be at full fee schedule allowable for CPT code 31578 for Medicare beneficiaries.

99   Multiple Modifiers

Under certain circumstances two or more modifiers may be necessary to completely delineate a service. In such situations modifier 99 should be added to the basic procedure, and the other applicable modifiers may be listed as part of the description of the service.

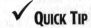

Quick Tip

Hospital ASC and Outpatient Coders
Medicare's instructions for modifiers 78 and 79 in hospital ASC or hospital outpatient facilities include in the definition procedures "return to the operating room on the same day." Use modifier 78 for a procedure related to the initial procedure on the same day and modifier 79 for a procedure on the same day that is unrelated to the initial procedure.

Key Point

When billing for an unrelated procedure by the same physician during the postoperative period of an original procedure, a new postoperative will begin with the subsequent procedure.

Using the Modifier Correctly
- If the third-party payer's computer system accepts multiple modifiers on the same line, then the 99 modifier is not needed. If the system does not, report modifier 99 as follows:
  —the 99 modifier is placed after a selected CPT code to illustrate to the payer that multiple modifiers apply to the service(s). Use modifier 99 on the basic service. Enter on the CMS-1500 claim form all applicable additional modifiers in item 19. If modifier 99 is entered on multiple line items, all applicable modifiers for each line item containing modifier 99 should be listed as follows: 1 = (mod), where the number "1" represents the specific line item and mod represents all modifiers applicable to the referenced line item. For electronic submissions, the additional modifiers should be listed in the extra narrative field, record HAO, field 05.0, positions 40 through 320. If the individual modifiers are not identified, the claim may be denied.

Incorrect Use of the Modifier
- Applying modifier 99 to a code with either one additional or no additional modifiers.

Coding Tips
- Modifier 99 is added to the basic service when more than two modifiers are needed to describe a service. The additional modifiers should be included with the claim (item 19 on paper claim submissions, or in the appropriate message free-form area on electronic submissions).
- Before using modifier 99, check with the third-party payers regarding their rules for its use.
- CPT codes for use with modifier 99 are 10021–69990, 70010–79999, and 90281–99600, when appropriate unless limited by the payer.

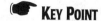

KEY POINT

Submitting 99 by Electronic Claims:
When submitting modifier 99, multiple modifiers, by electronic claims, many third-party payers, including some Medicare carriers, require the modifier 99 in the first modifier field, the second modifier in the second modifier field, and the remaining modifiers in the narrative (HAO) record.

When submitting only two modifiers or less and, therefore, not reporting the modifier 99, continue to use only the first and second modifier fields.

Chapter 7: HCPCS Modifiers A-V

INTRODUCTION

The HCPCS Level II codes are alphanumeric codes developed by CMS as a complementary coding system to the AMA's CPT codes. HCPCS Level II codes describe procedures, services and supplies not found in the CPT manual.

Similar to the CPT coding system, HCPCS Level II codes also contain modifiers that serve to further define services and items without changing the basic meaning of the CPT or HCPCS Level II code with which they are reported. The HCPCS Level II modifiers differ somewhat from their CPT counterparts, however, in that they are composed of either alpha characters or alphanumeric characters. HCPCS Level II modifiers range from AA to VP, and include such diverse modifiers as E1 upper left, eyelid, GJ opt out physician or practitioner for emergency or urgent service, and Q6 service furnished by a locum tenens physician.

It is important to note that HCPCS Level II modifiers may be used in conjunction with CPT codes, such as 69436-LT, tympanostomy (requiring insertion of ventilating tube), general anesthesia, left ear. Likewise, CPT modifiers can be used when reporting HCPCS Level II codes, such as L4396-50. Ankle contracture splint, bilateral (this scenario can also be reported with the RT and LT modifiers, depending on the third-party payer's protocol). In some cases, a report may be required to accompany the claim to support the need for a particular modifier's use, especially in cases when the presence of a modifier causes suspension of the claim for manual review and pricing.

AMBULANCE MODIFIERS

For ambulance services modifiers, there are single alpha characters with distinct definitions that are paired together to form a two-character modifier. The first character indicates the origination of the patient (e.g., patient's home, physician office, etc.) and the second character indicates the destination of the patient (e.g., hospital, skilled nursing facility, etc.). When reporting ambulance services, the name of the hospital or facility should be included on the claim(s). If reporting the scene of an accident or acute event (character S) as the origin of the patient, a written description of the actual location of the scene or event must be included with the claim(s).

D   Diagnostic or therapeutic site/free standing facility (i.e., dialysis center, radiation therapy center) other than "P" or "H"

E   Residential or domiciliary/custodial facility (i.e., nonskilled facility)

G   Hospital-based dialysis facility (hospital or hospital-associated)

©2003 Ingenix, Inc.
CPT only ©2003 American Medical Association. All Rights Reserved.

H Hospital-inpatient/outpatient (does not include an attached nursing facility or swing-bed; use "N" instead)

I Site of transfer (e.g., airport or helicopter pad) between modes of transfer

J Nonhospital based dialysis facility

N Skilled nursing facility (includes swing-bed)

P Physician office

R Private residence

S Scene of accident or acute event

X (Destination code only), intermediate stop at physician's office on the way to the hospital

HCPCS LEVEL II MODIFIERS

Alphabetical Listing

A1 Dressing for one wound

A2 Dressing for two wounds

A3 Dressing for three wounds

A4 Dressing for four wounds

A5 Dressing for five wounds

A6 Dressing for six wounds

A7 Dressing for seven wounds

A8 Dressing for eight wounds

A9 Dressing for nine or more wounds

AA Anesthesia performed personally by anesthesiologist
- CPT codes approved for use of the -AA modifier are 00100–01999.
- If an anesthetist assists the physician in the care of a single patient, the service is considered personally performed by the physician. The anesthesiologist should report this service with the AA modifier and the appropriate CPT code from series 00100–01999.
- Modifier AA affects Medicare payment.

AD Medical supervision by a physician; more than four concurrent anesthesia procedures
- Modifier AD affects Medicare payment as a distinct fee schedule amount exists.

AH Clinical psychologist

AJ Clinical social worker
- Medicare limits allowable to 75 percent of the physician fee schedule.

AM Physician, team member service

Chapter 7: HCPCS Modifiers A-V

- The physician member of a team is required to perform one out of every three visits made by a team member.
- The AM modifier should be used to indicate a team member visit was performed by the physician.
- Team member visits will be denied if only one person rendering services is billing for team services, as this is inappropriate billing practice.
- Modifier AM has no effect on payment.

AP Determination of refractive state was not performed in the course of diagnostic ophthalmological examination
- Modifier AP has no effect on payment.

AS Physician assistant, nurse practitioner or clinical nurse specialist services for assistant-at-surgery

AT Acute treatment
- This modifier should be used when reporting services 98940, 98941, or 98942.
- Modifier AT has no effect on payment for Medicare and many third-party carrier claims.

AU Item furnished in conjunction with a urological, ostomy, or tracheostomy supply

AV Item furnished in conjunction with a prosthetic device, prosthetic, or orthotic

AW Item furnished in conjunction with a surgical dressing

AX Item furnished in conjunction with dialysis services

BA Item furnished in conjunction with parenteral enteral nutrition (PEN) services

BO Orally administered nutrition, not by feeding tube

BP The beneficiary has been informed of the purchase and rental options and has elected to purchase the item

BR The beneficiary has been informed of the purchase and rental options and has elected to rent the item

BU The beneficiary has been informed of the purchase and rental options and after 30 days has not informed the supplier of his/her decision

CA Procedure payable only in the inpatient setting when performed emergently on an outpatient who expires prior to admission

CB Service ordered by a renal dialysis facility (RDF) physician as part of the esrd beneficiary's dialysis benefit, is not part of the composite rate, and is separately reimbursable

CC Procedure code change
- Modifier CC is used by the carrier when the procedure code submitted had to be changed either for administrative reasons or because an incorrect code was filed.
- Payment rule: Payment determination will be based on the new code used by the carrier.
- Modifier CC has no effect on payment.

©2003 Ingenix, Inc.
CPT only ©2003 American Medical Association. All Rights Reserved.

Ingenix Coding Lab: Understanding Modifiers

E1   Upper left, eyelid

E2   Lower left, eyelid

E3   Upper right, eyelid

E4   Lower right, eyelid

EJ   Subsequent claims for a defined course of therapy (e.g., EPO, sodium)

EM   Emergency reserve supply (for ESRD benefit only)

EP   Service provided as part of Medicaid Early Periodic Screening Diagnosis and Treatment (EPSDT) program

ET   Emergency treatment
- This modifier should be applied to report dental procedures performed in emergency situations.

EY   No physician or other licensed health care provider order for this item or service

F1   Left hand, second digit

F2   Left hand, third digit

F3   Left hand, fourth digit

F4   Left hand, fifth digit

F5   Right hand, thumb

F6   Right hand, second digit

F7   Right hand, third digit

F8   Right hand, fourth digit

F9   Right hand, fifth digit

FA   Left hand, thumb

FP   Service provided as part of Medicaid family planning program

G1   Most recent URR reading of less than 60
- URR is the urea reduction ratio, a calculation that demonstrates the effectiveness of renal dialysis.

G2   Most recent URR reading of 60 to 64.9

G3   Most recent URR reading of 65 to 69.9

G4   Most recent URR reading of 70 to 74.9

G5   Most recent URR reading of 75 or greater

G6   ESRD patient for whom less than six dialysis sessions have been provided in a month
- The Balanced Budget Act (BBA) of 1997 requires CMS to develop and implement a method to measure and report on the quality of dialysis services.

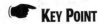

KEY POINT

Modifier 59 was established (and replaced the HCPCS Level II modifier GB, deleted in 1997) to demonstrate that multiple yet distinct services were provided to a patient on the same date of service by the same provider. Because distinct procedures or services rendered on the same day by the same physician cannot be easily identified and therefore properly adjudicated by simply listing the CPT procedure codes, modifier 59 assists the third-party payer or Medicare carrier in applying the appropriate reimbursement protocol. If the modifier is not used in these circumstances, a denial of services may ensue, with the explanation of benefits stating, for instance for Medicare claims, "Medicare does not pay for this service because it is part of another service that was performed at the same time."

Chapter 7: HCPCS Modifiers A-V

- ESRD facilities must use modifiers on or after January 1, 1998, to reflect the most recent urea reduction ratio (URR), along with CPT code 90999, unlisted dialysis procedure inpatient or outpatient, on all claims filed to Medicare for hemodialysis. Consequently, it will be necessary for ESRD facilities to also report a HCPCS code with the dialysis revenue code (820, 821, and 829). ESRD facilities (both hospital-based and free-standing) should report CPT code 90999 and one of the G modifiers as appropriate, on all claims filed for hemodialysis services on or after January 1, 1998. This information will provide data to CMS regarding the adequacy of hemodialysis for quality improvement initiatives. ESRD facilities must monitor hemodialysis adequacy monthly for all facility patients. Home hemodialysis patients may be monitored less frequently, but not less often than quarterly.

- Because CMS will be profiling facilities based on the URR ranges reported, CMS is recommending dialysis facilities to use a standardized methodology for drawing the pre- and postdialysis blood urea nitrogen (BUN) samples that are used in the calculation of the URR. Facilities may use either the slow flow/stop pump or blood reinfusing sampling techniques.

G7   The pregnancy resulted from rape or incest, or pregnancy certified by physician as life threatening

- This modifier is appended to the CPT procedure code(s) for abortion services and indicates that the pregnancy resulted from rape or incest, or that the physician considers the pregnancy to be life threatening to the mother.

- Reporting this modifier on a claim communicates to the carrier that the physician certifies that the abortion meets Medicare's coverage policy. Medicare will cover an abortion when:

  the pregnancy is the result of an act of rape or incest

  the woman suffers from a physical disorder, physical injury or physical illness, including a life-endangering physical condition caused by or arising from the pregnancy itself, that would, as certified by a physician, place the woman in danger of death unless an abortion is performed

- Claims submitted with modifier G7 for abortion services may be subject to postpayment review by the carrier.

- Third-party payers, other than Medicare, may not accept this modifier. Individual payers should be queried for claim submission requirements.

G8   Monitored anesthesia care (MAC) for deep complex, complicated or markedly invasive surgical procedure

G9   Monitored anesthesia care for patient who has a history of severe cardio-pulminary condition

GA   Waiver of liability statement on file

- This modifier indicates that the physician's office has a signed advance beneficiary notice (ABN) retained in the patient's chart.

- The purpose of the waiver of liability is to ensure that the provider will be paid for the services performed, and to protect the beneficiary from receiving unnecessary services. Providers who acquire a waiver of liability for a service should use the GA modifier directly following a procedure code to indicate that a beneficiary has signed a waiver of liability form. The provider should keep the form on file. No other statement regarding the waiver of liability is required when the GA modifier is used. Modifier GA at the end of a procedure code is sufficient

---

©2003 Ingenix, Inc.
CPT only ©2003 American Medical Association. All Rights Reserved.

117

Ingenix Coding Lab: Understanding Modifiers

evidence that the beneficiary has signed an advance notice and has agreed to pay for the service in the event it is denied as not medically necessary by Medicare. If the beneficiary subsequently requests a review of the denial, Medicare will request the physician to forward a copy of the notice for their files.

- An important preventive measure that the physician can use to avoid most claim denials when the services are medically reasonable and necessary, is to fully complete their claims. Medical necessity denials are often due to a lack of information on the claim to support the medical necessity of the service.
- An advanced notice may be applied to an extended course of treatment provided the notice identifies each service for which Medicare is likely to deny payment. A separate notice is required, however, if additional services for which Medicare is likely to deny payment are furnished later in the course of treatment.
- The Medicare beneficiary is never liable for payment of services that are unbundled from another service. Examples of unbundled services include two hospital visits on the same day by the same physician, removal of sutures by the same physician who performed the surgical procedure, and administration of an injection on the day of an evaluation and management service.
- Modifier GA has no effect on payment; however, potential liability determinations are based, in part, on the use of this modifier.

GB Claim being resubmitted for payment because it is no longer covered under a global payment demonstration

GC This service has been performed in part by a resident under the direction of a teaching physician
- When a teaching physician's services are billed using this modifier, the teaching physician is certifying that he or she was present during the key portion(s) of the service and was immediately available during the other portions of the service.
- When an anesthesiologist uses modifier QK for two to four medically directed procedures, he or she would not also append modifier GC to the anesthesia code. modifier QK only is used.
- When there is a one-on-one situation with a resident and a teaching anesthesiologist (teaching setting) the anesthesiologist would append modifier GC only.
- The QK and the GC modifiers are never used together.
- Modifier GC has no effect on payment.

GE This service has been performed by a resident without the presence of a teaching physician under the primary care exemption
- This modifier identifies services being billed under the primary care exception to the guideline for governing presence during the key portion(s) of a service by the teaching physician.
- Modifier GE has no effect on payment.

GF Nonphysician (e.g. nurse practitioner (NP), certified registered nurse anaesthetist (CRNA), certified registered nurse (CRN), clinical nurse specialist (CNS), physician assistant (PA)) services in a critical access hospital

GG As of January 1, 2002, Medicare issued new billing instructions when additional films are ordered when a radiologist interpretation of a screening mammogram results in an additional diagnostic mammogram. Modifier GG will be required to be appended to the claim for the diagnostic mammogram,

KEY POINT

The HCPCS Level II modifier GH became effective for dates of services on or after October 1, 1998. The Medicare program, with the reporting of this modifier, will allow a radiologist to order additional views of the mammogram study when the original views show signs of an abnormality or potential problem. When additional mammography views are ordered, the study changes from a screening to a diagnostic study. This can be accomplished by the radiologist without the consent of the ordering or treating physician.

Chapter 7: HCPCS Modifiers A-V

thus allowing the screening (CPT 76092) and diagnostic (CPT 76090 or CPT 76091) films to be paid. Modifier GH will still be required when a screening mammogram is converted to a diagnostic mammogram (screening mammogram will not be billed).

GH Diagnostic mammogram converted from screening mammogram on same day
- Report CPT code 76092 for a screening mammogram; however, if the study is converted to a diagnostic mammogram by the ordering of additional view(s) to rule out or to better visualize a suspected abnormality seen on the screening view(s), then report CPT code 76090 appended with modifier GH.
- The radiologist is considered the ordering physician in this situation and must furnish his/her unique physician identification number (UPIN) for Medicare claims. Diagnostic mammography claims submitted to Medicare without the ordering physician's UPIN will be denied and returned as unprocessable.

GJ Opt Out physician or practitioner emergency or urgent service
- Use this modifier for claims submitted to Medicare for services rendered by an opt out provider who has not signed a private contract with the Medicare patient requiring either emergent or urgent medical care.
- The provider may not charge the Medicare beneficiary more than what a non-participating provider would be permitted to charge, and must submit the claim to Medicare on the beneficiary's behalf.
- If modifier GJ is not reported on the claim for emergency or urgent care rendered to a Medicare beneficiary by the opt out provider, the claim will be denied and returned as unprocessable.

GK Actual item/service ordered by physician, item associated with GA or GZ modifier

GL Medically unnecessary upgrade provided instead of standard item. No charge. No advance beneficiary notice.

GM Multiple patients on one ambulance trip

GN Service delivered under an outpatient speech-language pathology plan of care

GO Service delivered under an outpatient occupational therapy plan of care

GP Service delivered under an outpatient physical therapy plan of care

GQ Via asynchronous telecommunications system

GT Via interactive audio and video telecommunication systems

GU Procedure performed in non fee schedule place of service

GV Attending physician not employed or paid under arrangement by the patient's hospice provider.

GW Service not related to hospice patient's terminal condition

GY Item or service statutorily excluded or does not meet the definition of any Medicare benefit.

GZ Item or service expected to be denied as not reasonable and necessary.

H9 Court-ordered

©2003 Ingenix, Inc.
CPT only ©2003 American Medical Association. All Rights Reserved.

Ingenix Coding Lab: Understanding Modifiers

HA Child/adolescent program

HB Adult program, non-geriatric

HC Adult program, geriatric

HD Pregnant/parenting women's program

HE Mental health program

HF Substance abuse program

HG Opioid addiction treatment program

HH Integrated mental health/substance abuse program

HI Integrated mental health and mental retardation/developmental disabilities program

HJ Employee assistance program

HK Specialized mental health programs for high-risk populations

HL Intern

HM Less than bachelor degree level

HN Bachelors degree level

HO Masters degree level

HP Doctoral level

HQ Group setting

HR Family/couple with client present

HS Family/couple without client present

HT Multi-disciplinary team

HU Funded by child welfare agency

HV Funded state addictions agency

HW Funded by state mental health agency

HX Funded by county/local agency

HY Funded by juvenile justice agency

HZ Funded by criminal justice agency

JW Drug amount discarded/not administered to any patient

K0 Lower extremity prosthesis functional level = 0; does not have the ability or potential to ambulate or transfer safely with or without assistance and a prosthesis does not enhance their quality of life or mobility

©2003 Ingenix, Inc.
CPT only ©2003 American Medical Association. All Rights Reserved.

Chapter 7: HCPCS Modifiers A-V

K1   Lower extremity prosthesis functional level = 1: has the ability or potential to use a prosthesis for transfers or ambulation on level surfaces at fixed cadence. Typical of the limited and unlimited household ambulator

K2   Lower extremity prosthesis functional level = 2: has the ability or potential for ambulation with the ability to traverse low level environmental barriers such as curbs, stairs or uneven surfaces. Typical of limited community ambulator

K3   Lower extremity prosthesis functional level = 3: has the ability or potential for ambulation with variable cadence. Typical of community ambulator who has the ability to traverse most environmental barriers and may have vocational, therapeutic or exercise activity that demands prosthetic utilization beyond simple locomotion

K4   Lower extremity prosthesis functional level = 4: has the ability or potential for prosthetic ambulation that exceeds the basic ambulation skills, exhibiting high impact, stress or energy levels, typical of the prosthetic demands of the child, active adult, or athlete

KA   Add-on option/accessory for wheelchair

KB   Beneficiary requested upgrade for abnormal, more than 4 modifiers identified on claim

KH   DMEPOS item, initial claim, purchase or first month rental
  • DMEPOS is the acronym for durable medical equipment, prosthetics, orthotics, and supplies
  • Report with modifier RR for rented DME.

KI   DMEPOS item, second or third month rental
  • Report with modifier RR for rented DME.

KJ   DMEPOS item, parenteral/enteral nutrition (PEN) pump or capped rental, months four to 15
  • Standard hospital beds are billed with HCPCS Level II codes E0250–E0266 or E0290–E0297. Hospital beds with a mattress that is wider than 36 inches and that can support a patient weighing more than 300 pounds must be submitted using code E1399, durable medical equipment, miscellaneous.
  • These beds are considered capped rental and, therefore, payment will only be made on a rental basis. The appropriate modifier (KH, KI, KJ) must be used and the rent/purchase option must be offered in the tenth rental month, as with all capped rental items.
  • Report with modifier RR for rented DME.

KM   Replacement of facial prosthesis including new impression/moulage

KN   Replacement of facial prosthesis using previous master model

KO   Single drug unit dose formulation

KP   First drug of a multiple drug unit dose formulation

KQ   Second or subsequent drug of a multiple drug unit formulation

KR   Rental item–billing for partial month

©2003 Ingenix, Inc.
CPT only ©2003 American Medical Association. All Rights Reserved.

121

Ingenix Coding Lab: Understanding Modifiers

KS Glucose monitor supply for diabetic beneficiary not treated with insulin

KX Specific required documentation on file

LC: Left circumflex coronary artery;

LD: Left anterior descending coronary artery; RC: Right coronary artery
- These codes are used when more than one intervention is required on a major vessel and its branches. CPT codes describe codes for coronary angioplasty, atherectomy and stent procedures in terms of the "initial" vessel and a "subsequent" vessel.
- These modifiers will be used to indicate the specific vessel involved in the procedure and should be used when one of the following procedures is reported:

92980: Transcatheter placement of an intracoronary stent(s), percutaneous, with or without other therapeutic intervention, any method; single vessel

92981: Each additional vessel (add-on code)

92982: Percutaneous transluminal coronary balloon angioplasty; single vessel

92984: Each additional vessel (add-on code)

92995: Percutaneous transluminal coronary atherectomy, by mechanical or other method, with or without balloon angioplasty; single vessel

92996: Each additional vessel (add-on code)

Note: Do not bill additional vessel codes without first billing the single vessel code.

- There are three procedures (stent, balloon angioplasty and atherectomy). Each procedure has two codes; a single vessel code and an additional vessel code. The single-vessel code is only used the first time that intervention is used during the interventional session. If the intervention is performed on more than one vessel, the additional vessel code(s) should be used. The following are examples of the proper way to code the vessels:

92980 RC, 92981 LC, 92981 LD
92980 RC, 92982 LC*, 92995 LD*
92982 RC, 92984 LC, 92984 LD
92995 RC, 92996 LC, 92996 LD
92995 RC, 92996 LC, 92982 LD*

- Procedure codes 92982 and 92995 cannot be billed separately from procedure code 92980 when provided on the same vessel. Procedure code 92982 cannot be billed separately from procedure code 92995 when performed on the same vessel. According to the CCI, the 59 modifier does not need to be included with these procedures.

LL Lease/rental (applied to purchase)
- Use this modifier when the DME rental amount is to be applied against the final purchase price of the DME.

LR Laboratory round trip

LS FDA-monitored intraocular lens implant

LT Left side

KEY POINT

HCPCS Level II modifiers may be used in conjunction with CPT codes, and vice versa.

CPT code-HCPCS Level II modifier combination: 69436-RT, tympanostomy (requiring insertion of ventilating tube), general anesthesia, right ear

HCPCS Level II code-CPT modifier combination: L4396-50, ankle contracture splint, bilateral (this scenario can also be reported with the RT and LT modifiers, depending on the third-party payer's protocol).*

Chapter 7: HCPCS Modifiers A-V

- This modifier indicates that side of the body on which a procedure is performed. It does not indicate a bilateral procedure. Lesion removal on the right arm and left arms should be coded with modifiers RT and LT.
- Lacrimal punctum plugs are used to close the puncta located at the inner corners of the eyes. Procedure code 68761 identifies the closure of a single punctum. In situations where two puncta are treated in the same eye (RT or LT, whichever applies), the physician should then bill 68761 (RT or LT) on the first line and 68761 (RT or LT) with modifier 76 on the next line.
- Modifiers LT and RT have no effect on payment; however, failure to use when appropriate could result in delay or denial (or partial denial) of the claim.

MS   Six-month maintenance and servicing fee for reasonable and necessary parts and labor, which are not covered under any manufacturer or supplier warranty

NR   New when rented (DME)
- Use this modifier when the DME, which was new at the time of its rental, is subsequently purchased.

NU   New equipment

PL   Progressive additional lenses

Q2   CMS/ORD demonstration project procedure/service

Q3   Live kidney donor: surgery and related services
- Use the Q3 modifier to identify postoperative live kidney donor services which are reimbursed at 100 percent of the Medicare fee schedule amount.

Q4   Service for ordering/referring physician qualifies as a service exemption
- Use this modifier when the ordering or referring provider has a financial relationship with the entity performing the service, and for which the service qualifies as one of the service-related exemptions.

Q5   Service performed by a substitute physician under a reciprocal billing arrangement
- Modifier Q5 is to be applied to the end of a procedure code to indicate that the service was provided by a substitute physician. The regular physician should keep a record on file of each service provided by the substitute physician, associated with the substitute physician's UPIN and make this record available to Medicare upon request.
- This modifier has no effect on payment.

Q6   Service furnished by a locum tenens physician
- A locum tenens physician generally has no practice of his or her own; they usually move from area to area as needed. The patient's regular physician may submit a claim and receive Medicare Part B payment for a covered and medically necessary visit of a locum tenens physician who is not an employee of the regular physician and whose services for patients of the regular physician are not restricted to the regular physician's office. The locum tenens physician should not provide the visit services to Medicare patients for a continuous period of longer than 60 days.
- This modifier has no effect on payment.

✓ QUICK TIP

CMS states fraud occurs when a person knowingly and willfully deceives the Medicare program or misrepresents information to obtain the benefit of monetary value, resulting in unauthorized Medicare payment to themselves or to another party.

The violator may be a participating or non-participating provider, a supplier of medical equipment, a Medicare beneficiary, or even an individual or business entity unrelated to a beneficiary. Defrauding the Medicare program of federal monies includes, but is not limited to, the following practices:

- Billing for services or supplies that were not provided (this includes billing the Medicare program for no show patients)
- Altering claim forms to obtain higher payment amounts
- Deliberately submitting claims for duplicate payment
- Soliciting, offering, or receiving a kickback, bribe, or rebate (common examples of this practices are:
  —paying an individual or business entity for the referral of a patient
  —routinely waiving a beneficiary's deductible and/or coinsurance
- Providing falsified certification of medical necessity (CMN) forms for patients not professionally known by the physician or supplier, or a supplier completing a CMN for the physician (ordering medical equipment and/or supplies not originating from the physician's orders)
- Falsely representing the nature, level, or number of services rendered or the identity of the beneficiary, dates of service, etc. (this includes billing a telephone call as if it were an actual patient visit)
- Collusion between a provider and a beneficiary or supplier resulting in higher costs or unnecessary charges to the Medicare program
- Using another person's Medicare card to authorize services for a different beneficiary or non-Medicare patient
- Altering claims history records to generate fraudulent payment
- Repeatedly violating the assignment agreement and/or limiting charge amounts
- Falsely representing provider ownership in a clinical laboratory
- Unauthorized use of the Medicare program's name or logo (a person may use neither the Medicare program's name nor logo, and cannot use the Social Security emblem in advertising for items or services as Medicare approved

---

©2003 Ingenix, Inc.
CPT only ©2003 American Medical Association. All Rights Reserved.

Q7, Q8, and Q9—Foot care

- Documentation of the systemic conditions and class findings must be in the patient's record. The record must be maintained in the physician's office and available for medical review by the carrier. Documentation should indicate the course of treatment and length of treatment for infectious conditions. Documentation should include the affected toe(s), including the clinical evidence of mycosis, the manner in which and to what extent the nail(s) were debrided, and the antifungal agent used in the office note/progress note.
- In addition, a description of the qualifying symptoms should be documented
- Ambulatory patients must exhibit a marked limitation in ambulation, pain or secondary infection resulting from the thickening and dystrophy.
- Non-ambulatory patients must suffer from pain or secondary infection resulting from the thickening and dystrophy of the infected nail plate.
- Routine foot care is excluded from Medicare coverage.
- General diagnosis such as ASHD, circulatory problems, vascular disease and venous insufficiency are not sufficient to permit payment for routine foot care.

Q7   One Class A finding

- Class A findings: Nontraumatic amputation of foot or integral skeletal portions thereof.
- This modifier was established to allow the provider to report class findings without having to write a narrative description on the claim form or submit additional documentation with the claim. This modifier should be used in conjunction with foot care procedures (e.g., 11720, 11721) to indicate the severity of the patient's systemic condition and justify the medical necessity of a procedure that is usually denied as routine.

Q8   Two Class B findings

- Class B findings:

    absent posterior tibial pulse

    absent dorsalis pedis pulse

    advance trophic changes such as (three required):

    - hair growth (decrease or absence)
    - nail changes (thickening)
    - pigmentary changes (discoloration)
    - skin texture (thin, shiny)
    - skin color (rubor or redness)

- This modifier was established to allow the provider to report class findings without having to write a narrative description on the claim form or submit additional documentation with the claim. This modifier should be used with foot care procedures (e.g., 11720, 11721) to indicate the severity of the patient's systemic condition and to justify the medical necessity of a procedure that is usually denied as routine.

Q9   One Class B and two Class C findings

- Class C findings:

    claudication

    temperature changes (e.g., cold feet)

    edema

    paresthesia

    burning

This modifier was established to allow the provider to report class findings without having to write a narrative description on the claim form or submit additional documentation with the claim. This modifier should be used in conjunction with foot care procedures (e.g., 11720, 11721) to indicate the severity of the patient's systemic condition and to justify the medical necessity of a procedure that is usually denied as routine.

QA FDA investigational device exemption.
- The IDE project number must be included on the claim when modifier QA is billed.

QB Physician providing service in a rural HPSA.
- Physician services furnished in a health professional shortage area (HPSA) qualify for a quarterly incentive payment. Global surgical packages may also qualify for these payments. The following guidelines apply for the HPSA incentive payment:

  If the entire global surgical package is furnished in a HPSA, the procedure code for the surgery should be reported with the applicable HPSA procedure code modifier (i.e., QB or QU).

  If only a portion of the global surgical package is performed in a HPSA, only the portion that is furnished in the HPSA should be reported with the HPSA modifier.

- Only physician services are eligible for the HPSA incentive payment. Do not bill nonphysician services with the QB modifier.
- Modifier QB has no effect on individual claim payment but generates a quarterly bonus payment.

QC Single channel monitoring

QD Recording and storage in solid state memory by a digital recorder.
- No effect on payment.

QE Prescribed amount of oxygen is less than 1 liter per minute (LPM)

QF Prescribed amount of oxygen exceeds 4 liters per minute (LPM) and portable oxygen is prescribed.

QG Prescribed amount of oxygen is greater than 4 liters per minute (LPM).

QH Oxygen conserving device is being used with an oxygen delivery system.

QJ Services/items provided to a prisoner or patient in state or local custody, however the state or local government, as applicable, meets the requirements in 42 CFR 411.4 (b)

QK Medical direction of two, three or four concurrent anesthesia procedures involving qualified individuals
- Payment rule: Limits payment to 55 percent of the amount that would have been allowed if personally performed by a physician or nonsupervised CRNA.
- When an anesthesiologist uses the QK modifier for 2–4 medically directed procedures, he or she would not also append GC to the anesthesia code. Use QK only.

> ### ✔ QUICK TIP
>
> CMS defines abuse of the federal Medicare program as "incidents or practices of providers, physicians, or suppliers of services and equipment which are inconsistent with accepted sound practices." Although in many instances these incidents or practices cannot be considered blatantly fraudulent, in some cases these incidents or practices may directly or indirectly result in unnecessary costs to the federal Medicare program. One of the most prevalent kinds of abuse is over-utilization of medical and health care services.
>
> Abuse of federal monies supporting the Medicare program includes but is not limited to the following practices:
>
> - Excessive charges for services, procedures or supplies
> - Claims for services not medically necessary, or for services not medically necessary to the extent rendered (for instance, a panel of tests is ordered when based upon the patient's working diagnosis, only a few of the tests within the panel were actually necessary)
> - Breaches of assignment agreements resulting in beneficiaries being billed for disallowed amounts
> - Improper billing practices, such as when the provider exceeds the Medicare imposed limiting charge (115 percent of the Medicare allowed amount for nonparticipating providers and for all providers of certain other services)
> - The submission of claims to Medicare when another third-party payer, managed care organization or workers' compensation carrier is the primary payer
> - Charging the Medicare program higher fees for Medicare patients than those charged to other third-party payers for non-Medicare patients

©2003 Ingenix, Inc.
CPT only ©2003 American Medical Association. All Rights Reserved.

- When there is a one-on-one situation with a resident and a teaching anesthesiologist, (teaching setting) the anesthesiologist would append the GC modifier only.
- Never use the QK and the GC modifiers together.

QL Patient pronounced dead after ambulance called

QM Ambulance service provided under arrangement by a provider of services
- Modifiers QM and QN should be used when a patient has an inpatient status at one hospital and is transferred to another hospital or facility for tests or treatment and then is returned to the first hospital.
- This modifier is valid for Medicare; however, the service would be denied under Medicare Part B since it is considered a Medicare Part A expense.

QN Ambulance service furnished directly by a provider of services
- Modifiers QM and QN should be used when a patient has an inpatient status at one hospital and is transferred to another hospital or facility for tests or treatment, and then is returned to the first hospital.
- This modifier is valid for Medicare; however, the service would be denied under Medicare Part B since it is considered a Medicare Part A expense.

QP Documentation is on file showing that the laboratory test(s) was ordered individually or ordered as a CPT-recognized panel other than automated profile codes (80002–80019, G0058–G0060)
- Sufficient documentation would be the requisition form showing that the physician had individually ordered tests either by code or the corresponding code definition.
- The individual tests that constitute an organ or disease related CPT panel do not need to be ordered individually in order for the laboratory to use the QP modifier. The laboratory may bill using the CPT code for organ or disease oriented panel with modifier QP when the physician orders the components of the panel.
- CMS does not require laboratories to use this modifier, but some carriers strongly advise its use.

QQ Claim submitted with a written statement of intent

QS Monitored anesthesia care services
- Monitored anesthesia care (MAC) services will be closely watched to ensure medical necessity is documented. ICD-9-CM codes should accurately describe the condition requiring MAC anesthesia. CMS collects data for MAC, even though it is paid the same as general anesthesia. The anesthesiologist or CRNA monitors the patient's vital signs, furnishes the preanesthesia exam, prescribe the necessary anesthesia care, administers medications and furnishes required postoperative anesthesia care. Documentation must be very clear in the record as to the medical necessity for monitored anesthesia care.

QT Recording and storage on tape by an analog tape recorder.
- This modifier has no effect on payment.

QU Physician providing service in an urban HPSA
- Modifier QU has no effect on payment but generates a quarterly bonus payment.

QUICK TIP

Claims for many of the items and services listed in the HCPCS Level II codes are handled by four specialized carriers called durable medical equipment regional carriers, or DMERCs. Claims are processed by the DMERCs based on the Medicare beneficiary's permanent residence, and not based on the site of service where the durable medical equipment, prosthetics, orthotics, and supplies (DMEPOS) item was dispensed.

A beneficiary's permanent residence is defined as the address where the beneficiary resides for more than six months a year. For foreign claims only, the DMERC jurisdiction is based on the site of service where the DMEPOS item was dispensed.

QV Item or service provided as routine care in a Medicare qualifying clinical trial
- Modifier QV is to be reported with V70.7 as the primary diagnosis code for CMS-1500 claims (professional services) and as a secondary diagnosis code for UB-92 claims for facilities.

QW CLIA-waived test
- Modifier QW is to be used for all codes that were designated as waived tests after 1996. For codes approved prior to 1996, the existing codes should be used without the modifier.

QX CRNA service with medical direction by a physician
- Payment rule: Limits payment to 55 percent of the amount that would have been allowed if personally performed by a physician or nonsupervised CRNA.

QY Anesthesiologist medically directs one CRNA

QZ CRNA service without medical direction by a physician
- Payment rule: No effect on payment. Payment would be equal to the amount that would have been allowed if personally performed by a physician.

RC Right coronary artery

RP Replacement and repair to indicate replacement of DME, orthotic, and prosthetic devices, which have been in use for some time

RR DME rental
- Use this modifier in conjunction with the appropriate ìrentalî modifiers KH, KI, and KJ.
- The RR modifier is placed directly after the HCPCS Level II code for the DME followed by the appropriate rental modifier as above.

RT Right side
- There are many procedure codes that require a physician to indicate the side of the body on which a procedure was performed by using the RT and LT modifiers.
- When billing for a separately identifiable/unrelated surgical procedure performed during the postoperative period of another surgical procedure, procedure code modifiers RT (right) and LT (left) must be indicated on the claim as appropriate. In addition, modifier 79 (unrelated procedure or service by the same physician during the postoperative period) must be submitted on the subsequent claim.
- This modifier indicates the side of the body on which a procedure is performed. It does not indicate a bilateral procedure. Lesion removal on the right arm and left arms should be coded with modifiers RT and LT.
- Lacrimal punctum plugs are used to close the puncta located at the inner corners of the eyes. Procedure code 68761 identifies the closure of a single punctum. In situations where two puncta are treated in the same eye, the physician should bill 68761 (RT or LT) on the first line and 68761 (RT or LT) with modifier 76 on the next line.
- Modifiers LT and RT has no effect on payment; however, failure to use when appropriate could result in delay or denial (or partial denial) of the claim.

SA Nurse practitioner rendering service in collaboration with a physician

SB Nurse midwife

QUICK TIP

There are certain procedure codes that describe and represent only the technical component portion of a procedure or service. These codes are stand-alone procedure or service codes, identifying the technician's or the supplier's technical services. In most cases, there are other procedure or service codes that identify the professional component only, and codes that represent both the professional and technical components as complete procedures or services called global service codes. It is not necessary to report modifier TC with codes that aptly describe and represent only the technical component of a procedure or service.

SC Medically necessary service or supply

SD Services provided by registered nurse with specialized, highly technical home infusion training

SE State and/or federally-funded programs/services

SF Second opinion ordered by QIO
- Use this modifier when the second opinion is ordered or requested by QIO.
- For Medicare beneficiaries, when this modifier is reported the service is eligible for 100 percent reimbursement. The usual deductible and/or coinsurance amounts are not applied.

SG Ambulatory surgery center (ASC) facility service
- ASCs should apply the modifier SG on all ASC facility services they file to Medicare, except when charging for supplies, such as V2785, processing, preserving and transposting corneal tissue. It is not necessary for physicians who provide services at ASC facilities to apply the SG modifier.
- Payment for the ASC facility service for Medicare patients will be based on the appropriate APC taken from the ASC payment list upon release of the final rule.

SH Second concurrently administered infusion therapy

SJ Third or more concurrently administered infusion therapy

SK Member of high risk population (use only with codes for immunization)

SL State supplied vaccine

ST Related to trauma or injury

SU Procedure performed in physician's office (to denote use of facility and equipment)

SV Pharmaceuticals delivered to patient's home but not utilized

T1 Left foot, second digit

T2 Left foot, third digit

T3 Left foot, fourth digit

T4 Left foot, fifth digit

T5 Right foot, great toe

T6 Right foot, second digit

T7 Right foot, third digit

T8 Right foot, fourth digit

T9 Right foot, fifth digit

TA Left foot, great toe

TC Technical component

Quick Tip

When submitted claims for routine items and services furnished in qualifying clinical trials, the billing provider should include information in the beneficiary's medical record about the clinical trial such as the trial name, sponsor, and sponsor-assigned protocol number. This information should not be submitted with the claim but should be provided if requested for medical review. A copy of routine items and services should also be made available if requested for medical review activities.

Chapter 7: HCPCS Modifiers A-V

- To report only the technical component, bill modifier TC with the procedure code. The payment includes the practice expense and the malpractice expense.
- There are stand-alone procedure codes which describe technical component only codes (e.g., staff and equipment costs) of diagnostic tests. They also identify procedures that are covered only as diagnostic tests and, therefore, do not have a related professional component. Do not use modifier TC on these codes. Technical component services only are institutional and should not be billed separately by the physicians. However, portable x-ray suppliers only bill for the technical component and should use modifier TC.
- Payment rule: Payment is based solely on the technical value of each individual procedure.

TD   RN

TE   LPN/lVN

TF   Intermediate level of care

TG   Complex/high tech level of care

TH   Obstetrical treatment/services, prenatal or postpartum

TJ   Program group, child and/or adolescent

TK   Extra patient or passenger, non-ambulance

TL   Early intervention/individualized family service plan (IFSP)

TM   Individualized education program (IEP)

TN   Rural/outside providers' customary service area

TP   Medical transport, unloaded vehicle

TQ   Basic life support transport by a volunteer ambulance provider

TR   School-based individualized education program (IEP) services provided outside the public school district responsible for the student

TS   Follow-up service

TT   Individualized service provided to more than one patient in same setting

TU   Special payment rate, overtime

TV   Special payment rates, holidays/weekends

TW   Back-up equipment

U1   Medicaid level of care 1, as defined by each state

U2   Medicaid level of care 2, as defined by each state

U3   Medicaid level of care 3, as defined by each state

U4   Medicaid level of care 4, as defined by each state

U5   Medicaid level of care 5, as defined by each state

©2003 Ingenix, Inc.
CPT only ©2003 American Medical Association. All Rights Reserved.

U6 Medicaid level of care 6, as defined by each state

U7 Medicaid level of care 7, as defined by each state

U8 Medicaid level of care 8, as defined by each state

U9 Medicaid level of care 9, as defined by each state

UA Medicaid level of care 10, as defined by each state

UB Medicaid level of care 11, as defined by each state

UC Medicaid level of care 12, as defined by each state

UD Medicaid level of care 13, as defined by each state

UE Used DME
   • Use this modifier when the used equipment is purchased by a beneficiary.

UF Services provided in the morning

UG Services provided in the afternoon

UH Services provided in the evening

UJ Services provided at night

UK Services provided on behalf of the client to someone other than the client

UN Two patients served

UP Three patients served

UQ Four patients served

UR Five patients served

US Six or more patients served

VP Aphakic patient
   • Modifier VP has no effect on payment

©2003 Ingenix, Inc.

CPT only ©2003 American Medical Association. All Rights Reserved.

Chapter 8: ASC and Hospital Outpatient Modifiers

AMBULATORY PAYMENT CLASSIFICATIONS

Following the implementation of Medicare's outpatient prospective payment system (OPPS), effective August 1, 2000, hospital outpatient services and provider-based clinics are reimbursed under the ambulatory payment classifications (APCs). The formulation of the APC grouping system took root in the ambulatory patient groups (APGs) system, devised by the Health Information Systems division of 3M Health Care under a grant from CMS. The APC reimbursement system for surgical procedures and other services; however, is not the same as the APG system (still in use by numerous payers).

The incorporation of APCs into each facility's internal coding and billing systems as well as clinical operations represents an enormous challenge. It is generally agreed that this system of reimbursement requires greater attention to operational economies and the creation of increased internal efficiencies when compared to the past implementation of the diagnosis-related group (DRG) system of reimbursement for the hospital inpatient arena.

CPT and certain HCPCS Level II codes map to a particular APC classification that holds a predefined reimbursement amount. The financial welfare of any facility outpatient (OP) department, OP clinic, hospital ambulatory surgery center (ASC), freestanding ASC, or private physician practice has always depended on the accurate coding and reporting of services. Now, with reimbursement for some of these health care centers based on the APCs system of reimbursement, the accurate coding and reporting of services has never been more critical. A few simple facts about APCs include the following:

- APCs are groups of services with homogenous or nearly-similar clinical characteristics as well as costs.
- At this time, APCs only affect hospital OP department/clinic and hospital ASC payment for Medicare patients.
- Physician payments are not affected.
- The APC payment system is correlated to the CPT and certain HCPCS Level II codes.
- Many CPT and HCPCS Level II codes map to an APC payment group.
- The encounter date for each patient may include one or more APC services.

The use of modifiers has proven to be a crucial component to the appropriate and optimal reimbursement of services by Medicare under APCs. Modifiers are addressed in the MIM, transmittal 1729, and the *Medicare Hospital Manual* (CMS Pub. 10), transmittal 726 (See CMS Web-based manual, pub 100-4, chapter 4). The modifier should be appended to the CPT/HCPCS Level-II procedure code. Each line item can hold two modifiers.

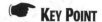 **KEY POINT**

Not all third-party payers will be using the new APC system of reimbursement for ASC and hospital outpatient facility services. There are several major third-party payers currently using (and seemingly satisfied with) the ambulatory patient groups (APGs) system of reimbursement for facility services.

Provider documentation has always been a critical aspect of appropriate reimbursement; however, under APCs the mandate for clear, concise, and complete medical record documentation, particularly in relation to modifier use, has never been stronger. Providers should be thoroughly debriefed about the immediate and long-term financial impact APCs will have on facilities and should be knowledgeable about the documentation requirements expected of them.

OUTPATIENT CODE EDITOR FOR OUTPATIENT PROSPECTIVE PAYMENT SYSTEM

Modifiers have proven to be a new territory of claims denials under the OPPS. The outpatient code editor (OCE) is a software package supplied to the fiscal intermediary (FI) by CMS to edit outpatient hospital claims. Prior to the OPPS implementation in August 2000, the OCE edited outpatient hospital claims to detect incorrect billing data and determine if the ASC limit should be applied to the claim. The OCE also reviewed each HCPCS and certain ICD-9-CM code for validity and coverage.

The OCE is updated quarterly and with each update comes new edits with claim delay reasons, claims processing instructions regarding discounting and modifiers, PRICER input information, Correct Coding Initiative (CCI) clarifications, units of service instructions, and other important updates. Maintaining a current version of the OCE for processing Medicare hospital claims is extremely important for hospital patient accounting departments.

In general, OCE performs all functions that require specific reference to HCPCS codes, HCPCS modifiers, and ICD-9-CM diagnosis codes. Since these coding systems are complex and updated annually, the centralization of the direct reference to these codes and modifiers in a single program will reduce effort for you and reduce the chance of inconsistent processing.

The header information passed to the OCE must relate to the entire claim and must include the following:

- From date
- Through date
- Condition code
- List of ICD-9-CM diagnosis codes
- Age
- Sex
- Type of bill
- Medicare provider number

The from and through dates will be used to determine if the claim spans more than one day and therefore represents multiple visits. The condition code (e.g., 41) specifies special claim conditions such as a claim for partial hospitalization, which is paid on a per diem basis. The diagnosis codes apply to the entire claim and are not specific to a line item.

Each line item contains the following information:

- HCPCS code with up to two modifiers

Chapter 8: ASC and Hospital Outpatient Modifiers

- Revenue code
- Service date
- Service units
- Charge

The HCPCS codes and modifiers are used as the basis of assigning the APCs.

There are currently 55 different edits in OCE, two of which are currently inactive. Each edit is assigned a number. The edit return buffers in the OCE consist of a list of the edit numbers that occurred for each diagnosis, procedure, modifier, or date.

The following modifier instructions were provided to providers as part of the OPPS implementation.

Modifier 25

Under some circumstances, medical visits on the same date as a procedure will result in additional payments. A modifier of 25 with an evaluation and management (E/M) (service indicator V) code is used to indicate that a medical visit was unrelated to any procedure that was performed with a type of T or S. E/M codes on the same day and same claim as a procedure of type T or S will have the medical APC assigned to all lines with E/M codes. However, if any E/M code that occurs on a claim with a type T or S procedure does not have a modifier of 25, then edit 21 will apply and there will be a line item rejection.

Discounting Modifiers

Line items with a service indicator of T are subject to multiple procedure discounting unless modifiers 76, 77, 78 and/or 79 are present. The line item with the highest payment amount will not be multiple procedure discounted, and all other T line items will be multiple procedure discounted. All line items that do not have a service indicator of T will be ignored in determining the discount. A modifier of 73 indicates that a procedure was terminated prior to anesthesia. A terminated procedure will also be discounted although not necessarily at the same level as the discount for multiple type T procedures. Terminated bilateral procedures or terminated procedures with units greater than one for type T procedures should not occur and have the discounting factor set so as to result in the equivalent of a single procedure. Bilateral procedures are identified from the "bilateral" field in the physician fee schedule. For non-type T procedures there is no terminated procedure or multiple bilateral discounting performed. Bilateral procedures have the following values in the "bilateral" field:

- Conditional bilateral (i.e., procedure is considered bilateral if the modifier 50 is present)
- Inherent bilateral (i.e., procedure in and of itself is bilateral)
- Independent bilateral (i.e., procedure is considered bilateral if the modifier 50 is present, but full payment should be made for each procedure, such as certain radiological procedures)

Inherent bilateral procedures will be treated as a non-bilateral procedure since the bilaterally of the procedure is encompassed in the code. For bilateral procedures the type T procedure discounting rules will take precedence over the discounting specified in the physician fee schedule. All line items for which the line item denial or

©2003 Ingenix, Inc.
CPT only ©2003 American Medical Association. All Rights Reserved.

133

reject indicator is 1 and the line item action flag is zero, or the line item action flag is 2 or 3, will be ignored in determining the discount.

The discounting process will utilize an APC payment amount file. The discounting factor for bilateral procedures is the same as the discounting factor for multiple type T procedures.

Other Modifier Reporting Requirements and Units of Service Restrictions

- The informational anatomic modifiers such as LT, RT, E1 through E4, FA, F1 through F9, TA, T1 through T9, LC, LD, RC should be used wherever appropriate to designate the anatomic site of a procedure performed. With the assumption that these modifiers are used whenever and wherever they are appropriate, the procedure codes to which these modifiers are allocated and applicable are assigned a unit of service equal to 1.

- Because of coding and payment instructions, the procedures to which modifier 50 (for bilateral procedure) are appended are assigned a unit of service equal to 1.

- In those instances where an anatomic or the bilateral modifier is not more appropriate, modifier 59 may be appropriate. On the first line, the code is reported without the modifier. On subsequent lines, the code is reported with modifier 59 and the unit of service is equal to 1. (In other words if a procedure is performed on three different sites, the first line will show the procedure code without the modifier, but with a unit of service of one. The next two lines will show the same procedure code, each with modifier 59 appended.)

- Where a procedure has to be repeated on the same anatomic site on the same day either by the same physician performing the first procedure (modifier 76) or by another physician (modifier 77), for the claim to be paid, the number of lines with the same code and modifier 76 or modifier 77 appended to all but the first code, must be less than, or equal to the maximum units allowed.

- The units of service edits for procedure codes submitted with modifier 91 (repeat clinical diagnostic laboratory test) do not apply. For clinical diagnostic laboratory tests, modifier 91 is appended to a code to indicate that the test was repeated on a different specimen. On the assumption that this modifier is used properly, no maximum units of service for procedures submitted with this modifier have been established. That is, procedures submitted with modifier 91 will bypass the units of service edits applied to clinical laboratory test codes in the 80000–89399 range of the CPT codes.

Correct Coding Initiative (CCI) Edits

Included in the OCE are over 65,000 of the CCI edits for code combination unbundling. These edits are similar to those developed for carrier processing; however, edits for anesthesiology, evaluation and management, mental health, critical care, and derma-bond edits have been removed. In addition, the carrier proprietary ("black box") edits have also not been included. Four of the OCE edits are related to appropriate modifier usage for CCI code combinations.

CCI edits in the OCE are always one quarter behind the carrier CCI edits. There are currently 55 different edits in the OCE, two of which are presently inactive. Each edit generated for a claim is associated with a disposition. The following table lists each edit related to modifier usage along with its respective claims disposition. Following is the table for the six claims dispositions applicable under OPPS.

Edit		Edit Type	Disposition
16.	Multiple bilateral procedures without modifier 50	Procedure edit	Claim returned to provider
17.	Inappropriate specification of bilateral procedure	Procedure edit	Claim returned to provider
19.	Mutually exclusive procedure that is not allowed by NCCI even if appropriate modifier is present	CCI, procedure edit	Line item rejection
20.	Component of a comprehensive procedure that is not allowed by NCCI even if appropriate modifier is present	CCI, procedure edit	Line item rejection
21.	Medical visit on same day as type T or S procedure without modifier 25	Procedure edit	Line item rejection
22.	Invalid modifier	Modifier edit	Claim returned to provider
39.	Mutually exclusive procedure that would be allowed by NCCI if appropriate modifier were present	CCI, procedure edit	Line item rejection
40.	Component of a comprehensive procedure that would be allowed by NCCI if appropriate modifier were present	CCI, procedure edit	Line item rejection

Disposition	Explanation
Claim rejection	Whole claim rejection. The provider can correct and resubmit the claim but cannot appeal the rejection.
Claim denial	Whole claim denial. The provider can not resubmit the claim but can appeal the denial.
Claim return to provider (RTP)	Whole claim returned to provider. The provider can resubmit the claim once the problems are corrected.
Claim suspension	Whole claim to be suspended. The claim is not returned to the provider, but it is not processed for payment until the fiscal intermediary makes a determination or obtains further information.
Line item rejection	One or more individual line items to be rejected. The claim can be processed for payment with some line items rejected for payment (i.e., the line item can be corrected and resubmitted but cannot be appealed).
Line item denial	One or more individual line items denied. The claim can be processed for payment with some line items denied for payment (i.e., the line item can not be resubmitted but can be appealed).

CPT AND HCPCS MODIFIER REPORTING REQUIREMENTS

With the release of the AMA's 1999 CPT code book, a new section containing modifiers for facility reporting was added. This section is continued in CPT 2004 and is found in appendix A, "Modifiers." These modifiers are to be reported for ASC and hospital outpatient services when appropriate. The AMA added a new modifier to the section of the appendix A for ASC and hospital outpatient reporting: 27, multiple outpatient hospital E/M encounters on the same date. Effective for services on or after October 1, 2001, Medicare will recognize and accept the use of modifier

©2003 Ingenix, Inc.
CPT only ©2003 American Medical Association. All Rights Reserved.

27. Note: This modifier will not replace the use of condition code G0 to indicate multiple outpatient hospital evaluation and management encounters on the same date.

Note: Check with Medicare and other third-party payers to ensure their recognition and acceptance of the following modifiers prior to reporting the modifiers on claims.

CPT Modifier	Description
25	Significant Separately Identifiable Evaluation and Management Service by the Same Physician on the Same Day of the Procedure or Other Service
27	Multiple Outpatient Hospital E/M Encounters on the Same Date
50	Bilateral Procedure
52	Reduced Services
58	Staged or Related Procedure or Service by the Same Physician During the Postoperative Period
59	Distinct Procedural Service
73	Discontinued Outpatient Hospital/ASC Procedure Prior to the Administration of Anesthesia
74	Discontinued Outpatient Hospital/ASC Procedure after Administration of Anesthesia
76	Repeat Procedure by Same Physician
77	Repeat Procedure by Another Physician
78	Return to the Operating Room for a Related Procedure During the Postoperative Period
79	Unrelated Procedure or Service by the Same Physician During the Postoperative Period
91	Repeat Clinical Diagnostic Laboratory Test

HCPCS Modifier	Description
LT	Left side
RT	Right side
E1	Upper left, eyelid
E2	Lower left, eyelid
E3	Upper right, eyelid
E4	Lower right, eyelid
FA	Left hand, thumb
F1	Left hand, second digit
F2	Left hand, third digit
F3	Left hand, fourth digit
F4	Left hand, fifth digit
F5	Right hand, thumb
F6	Right hand, second digit
F7	Right hand, third digit
F8	Right hand, fourth digit
F9	Right hand, fifth digit
GG	Performance and payment of a screening mammogram and diagnostic mammogram on the same patient, same day

Chapter 8: ASC and Hospital Outpatient Modifiers

HCPCS Modifier	Description
GH	Diagnostic mammogram converted from screening mammogram on same day
TA	Left foot, great toe
T1	Left foot, second digit
T2	Left foot, third digit
T3	Left foot, fourth digit
T4	Left foot, fifth digit
T5	Right foot, great toe
T6	Right foot, second digit
T7	Right foot, third digit
T8	Right foot, fourth digit
T9	Right foot, fifth digit
LC	Left circumflex coronary artery
LD	Left anterior descending coronary artery
RC	Right coronary artery
QM	Ambulance service provided under arrangement by a provider of services
QN	Ambulance service furnished directly by a provider of services

Coding Tips

- As of July 1, 1998, per hospital transmittal number 726, and subsequent related transmittals CMS requires CPT and HCPCS Level II modifiers to be reported for accuracy in reimbursement, coding consistency, editing and capture of payment data.
- The appropriate modifier is appended to the CPT procedure code to communicate that the code has been altered as indicated.
- To report terminated surgical procedures, whether before or after administration of anesthesia, see modifiers 73 and 74.

25 SIGNIFICANT SEPARATELY IDENTIFIABLE E/M SERVICE BY THE SAME PHYSICIAN ON THE SAME DAY OF THE PROCEDURE OR OTHER SERVICE

The physician may need to indicate that on the day a procedure or service identified by a CPT code was performed, the patient's condition required a significant, separately identifiable E/M service above and beyond the other service provided or beyond the usual preoperative and postoperative care associated with the procedure that was performed. The E/M service may be prompted by the symptom or condition for which the procedure and/or service was provided. As such, different diagnoses are not required for reporting of the E/M services on the same date. This circumstance may be reported by adding the modifier 25 to the appropriate level of E/M service.

Note: This modifier is not used to report an E/M service that resulted in a decision to perform surgery. See modifier 57.

Coding Tips

- This modifier should be used when the E/M service is separate and distinct from any procedure or other service provided. A clearly documented E/M service that is significant and separately identifiable must be in evidence.

QUICK TIP

Hospital ASC and Outpatient Coders

Facilities should use 25 in place of modifier 57 for the emergency department visit on the same day as a procedure that has a status of indicator of S or T. Modifier 57 is not a valid hospital/ASC modifier.

Facilities should use 25 for an emergency department visit on the same day as a procedure that has a status of indicator of S or T per CMS transmittal A-01-80 to avoid an OCE edit. This edit, however, does not preclude the use of modifier 25 on E/M codes when they are reported with procedure codes that are assigned to other than S or T status indicators as long as the E/M meets the definition of a "significant, separately identifiable" service.

Modifier 25 should be appended on to E/M service codes within the range of 92002–92014, 99201–99499, and with HCPCS codes G0101 and G0175.

©2003 Ingenix, Inc.
CPT only ©2003 American Medical Association. All Rights Reserved.

- Modifier 25 can only be appended to E/M service codes.
- Medicare has stated that modifier 25 "may be appended to the emergency department (ED) E/M code (99281–99285) when provided on the same date as a diagnostic medical/surgical and/or therapeutic medical/surgical procedure(s)." The E/M service must meet the definition above.
- The diagnosis linked to the E/M service reported with modifier 25 does not need to be different from the ICD-9-CM code reported with the medical/surgical and/or therapeutic medical/surgical procedure(s) provided.
- When a patient receives E/M services in different hospital outpatient clinics on the same day (i.e., is evaluated in these disparate departments/clinics but medical/surgical and/or therapeutic medical/surgical procedure[s] are not provided), modifier 25 is not appropriate for reporting purposes; instead, modifier 27 is reported (see information for modifier 27 that follows).

27   Multiple Outpatient Hospital E/M Encounters on the Same Date

For hospital outpatient reporting purposes, utilization of hospital resources related to separate and distinct E/M encounters performed in multiple outpatient hospital settings on the same date may be reported by adding modifier 27 to each appropriate level outpatient and/or emergency department E/M code(s). This modifier provides a means of reporting circumstances involving evaluation and management services provided by physician(s) in more than one (multiple) outpatient hospital setting(s) (e.g., hospital emergency department, clinic). **Note:** This modifier is not to be used for physician reporting of multiple E/M services performed by the same physician on the same date. For physician reporting of all outpatient evaluation and management services provided by the same physician on the same date and performed in multiple outpatient setting(s) (e.g., hospital emergency department, clinic), see Evaluation and Management, Emergency Department, or Preventive Medicine Services codes.

Coding Tips
- This modifier was established to help resolve the reporting of hospital resources directly related to the provision of E/M encounters rendered on the same date in various outpatient hospital settings.
- Modifier 27 should be appended to the second and/or subsequent E/M codes.
- When a patient is evaluated in different hospital outpatient clinics on the same day, each clinic should report the appropriate level E/M code (in accordance with the particular E/M guidelines the facility has decided to establish to support its E/M reporting system until such time that CMS mandates a standardized E/M reporting structure for facilities). The 27 modifier should be applied.
- Generally, condition code G0 (G-zero) is to be reported to specifying federal and state payers when multiple E/M services are provided on the same day, as long as the services fall under the same revenue code. If, for example, an E/M service was provided to a patient in an outpatient clinic and later that same day in the ED, both E/M services should be reported, but condition code G0 would not be reported because of the difference in revenue codes involved. Modifier 27 should be applied.

Hospital ASC and Outpatient Coders
Modifier 27 should be appended on to E/M service codes within the range of 92002–92014, 99201–99499, and with HCPCS codes G0101 and G0175.

50 BILATERAL PROCEDURE

Unless otherwise identified in the listings, bilateral procedures that are performed at the same operative session should be identified by adding the modifier 50 to the appropriate five-digit code.

Coding Tips

- This modifier is used to report bilateral procedures that are performed at the same operative session.
- For Medicare claims, report the bilateral procedures with one procedure code appended with modifier 50. This should appear on the UB-92 form, CMS-1500 claim form or in the appropriate field for electronic claims as one-line item, with a unit number of one. However, many Medicare carriers will also accept bilateral procedures reported as two-line items with the right (RT) and left (LT) HCPCS Level II modifiers appended to the respective procedure codes.
- The intermediary will reject the following surgical procedures if they are reported with modifier 50:

    surgical procedures identified by their terminology as bilateral (e.g., 27395–Lengthening of hamstring tendon, multiple, bilateral)

    surgical procedures identified as unilateral or bilateral (e.g., 52290, cystourethroscopy, with ureteral meatotomy, unilateral, or bilateral).

52 REDUCED SERVICES

Under certain circumstances a service or procedure is partially reduced or eliminated at the physician's discretion. Under these circumstances the service provided can be identified by its usual procedure number and the addition of the modifier 52, signifying that the service is reduced. This provides a means of reporting reduced services without disturbing the identification of the basic service. **Note:** For hospital outpatient reporting of a previously scheduled procedure/service that is partially reduced or canceled as a result of extenuating circumstances or those that threaten the well-being of the patient prior to or after administration of anesthesia, see modifiers 73 and 74.

Coding Tips

- Modifier 52 is used to indicate that, under certain circumstances, a service or procedure is partially reduced or eliminated at the physician's discretion.
- The 52 modifier is for a reduced service and is not a modifier to be used in situations when the fee is reduced for a patient due to his or her inability to pay the full charge.
- Facilities reporting this modifier with a procedure code should ensure that modifier 73, representing a discontinued procedure prior to the administration of anesthesia, or modifier 74, representing a discontinued procedure following the administration of anesthesia, do not more aptly describe the service.
- Modifier 52 is used to report a procedure that has been performed at a lesser level, or a procedure that has accomplished less results than expected (as defined by the CPT code description).

Hospital ASC and Outpatient Coders

Per Medicare, modifier 52, reduced service, is used in the hospital outpatient department to identify a procedure not requiring anesthesia (meaning general, regional, or local) that was terminated after the patient was prepared for the procedure (including any sedation). Reimbursement for modifier 52 procedures is 50 percent.

When a radiology procedure is reduced, the correct reporting is to code to the extent of the procedure performed. If no code exists for what has been done, report the intended code with modifier 52 appended.

Medicare's instructions for modifier 58 in hospital ASC or hospital outpatient facilities include in the definition procedures performed on the same calendar day.

58   Staged or Related Procedure or Service by the Same Physician During the Postoperative Period

The physician may need to indicate that the performance of a procedure or service during the postoperative period was: a) planned prospectively at the time of the original procedure (staged); b) more extensive than the original procedure; or c) for therapy following a diagnostic surgical procedure. This circumstance may be reported by adding the modifier 58 to the staged or related procedure. **Note:** This modifier is not used to report the treatment of a problem that requires a return to the operating room. See modifier 78.

Coding Tips

- Information on the application of this modifier, at this time, is consistent with the definition established by the AMA in CPT 2003. This modifier is reported when a second, staged/related procedure or service is performed during the postoperative period of another staged/related procedure.
- Do not confuse the application of this modifier with that of modifier 78, return to the operating room for a related procedure during a patient's postoperative period. While modifier 58 is reported when a staged/related procedure has been planned or is otherwise in agreement with the modifier's definition, modifier 78—though on the surface quite similar in definition—is reported for a related procedure performed that is unrelated and/or less extensive than the original procedure. (For unrelated procedures performed during the postoperative period, see modifier 79.)
- Do not report this modifier with procedures described as requiring multiple procedures. Procedures considered "multiple sessions" by definition are those that must be rendered at more than one service session.
- Medical record documentation should unambiguously establish the fact that staged/related procedures were performed.

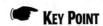

Key Point

Use modifier 59 only when the subsequent procedure occurs on the same date as another procedure by the same provider.

59   Distinct Procedural Service

Under certain circumstances, the physician may need to indicate that a procedure or service was distinct or independent from other services performed on the same day. Modifier 59 is used to identify procedures/services that are not normally reported together, but are appropriate under the circumstances. This may represent a different session or patient encounter, different procedure or surgery, different site or organ system, separate incision/excision, separate lesion, or separate injury (or area of injury in extensive injuries) not ordinarily encountered or performed on the same day by the same physician. However, when another already established modifier is appropriate it should be used rather than modifier 59. Only if a more descriptive modifier is not available, and the use of modifier 59 best explains the circumstances, should modifier 59 be used.

Coding Tips

- This modifier is used to identify procedures/services that are not normally reported together but may be performed under certain circumstances. This may represent a different session or patient encounter, different procedure or surgery, different site or organ system, separate incision or separate injury (or area of injury in extensive injuries) not ordinarily encountered or performed on the same day by the same physician.

Key Point

Modifier 59 was established (and replaced the HCPCS Level II modifier GB) to demonstrate that multiple yet distinct services were provided to a patient on the same date of service by the same provider. If this modifier is not used in these circumstances, a denial of services may ensue, with the explanation of benefits stating, for instance for Medicare claims, "Medicare does not pay for this service because it is part of another service that was performed at the same time."

- This modifier is used to indicate that a procedure or service was distinct or independent from other services performed on the same day.
- Append this modifier only to the procedure(s) considered distinct or independent from the other procedures performed or provided on the same day.
- Modifier 59 is only used when there is not another more descriptive modifier for the procedure or service.
- Modifier 59 is not reported with E/M codes.

73 DISCONTINUED OUTPATIENT HOSPITAL/AMBULATORY SURGERY CENTER (ASC) PROCEDURE PRIOR TO THE ADMINISTRATION OF ANESTHESIA

Due to extenuating circumstances or those that threaten the well-being of the patient, the physician may cancel a surgical or diagnostic procedure subsequent to the patient's surgical preparation (including sedation when provided, and being taken to the room where the procedure is to be performed), but prior to the administration of anesthesia (local, regional block(s) or general). Under these circumstances, the intended service that is prepared for but cancelled can be reported by its usual procedure number and the addition of the modifier 73. **Note:** The elective cancellation of a service prior to the administration of anesthesia and/or surgical preparation of the patient should not be reported. For physician reporting of a discontinued procedure, see modifier 3.

Coding Tips
- Use this modifier when the facility must report that services were discontinued following the physician's decision to discontinue the procedure due to extenuating circumstances or circumstances in which the well-being of the patient is threatened.
- Use this modifier when the patient has been surgically prepped but anesthesia has not been induced (local, regional or general).
- Report this modifier with the intended CPT procedure code(s) representing the discontinued service(s).

Hospital ASC and Outpatient Coders

Procedures reported with modifier 73 will receive 50 percent reimbursement under OPPS.

Modifier 53 is not applicable in hospital ASC or hospital outpatient facilities in accordance with CPT modifiers approved for ambulatory surgery center (ASC) outpatient hospital use.

74 DISCONTINUED OUTPATIENT HOSPITAL/AMBULATORY SURGERY CENTER (ASC) PROCEDURE AFTER ADMINISTRATION OF ANESTHESIA

Due to extenuating circumstances or those that threaten the well-being of the patient, the physician may terminate a surgical or diagnostic procedure after the administration of anesthesia (local, regional block(s), general) or after the procedure was started (incision made, intubation started, scope inserted, etc.). Under these circumstances, the procedure started, but terminated, can be reported by its usual procedure number and the addition of the modifier 74. **Note:** The elective cancellation of a service prior to the administration of anesthesia and/or surgical preparation of the patient should not be reported. For physician reporting of a discontinued procedure, see modifier 53.

Coding Tips
- Use this modifier when the facility must report that services were terminated at the physician's discretion due to extenuating circumstances, or circumstances in which the well-being of the patient is threatened.

Hospital ASC and Outpatient Coders

Procedures reported with modifier 74 will receive 100 percent reimbursement under OPPS.

Modifier 53 is not applicable in hospital ASC or hospital outpatient facilities in accordance with CPT modifiers approved for ambulatory surgery center (ASC) outpatient hospital use.

- Use this modifier when the patient has had anesthesia administered and/or induced (local, regional or general) or after the procedure was started including, but not limited to, one or more of the following services:

  intubation

  incision made

  scope inserted

76   REPEAT PROCEDURE BY SAME PHYSICIAN

The physician may need to indicate that a procedure or service was repeated subsequent to the original procedure or service. This circumstance may be reported by adding the modifier 76 to the repeated procedure/service.

Coding Tips

- This modifier is used to indicate that a procedure or service was repeated in a separate operative session, on the same day and does not represent a duplicate billing.
- When the procedure is repeated on the same day, the procedure code is reported once and then report it again with the modifier 76 added (two line items).
- If the third-party payer requires a one line item only reporting of a procedure repeated on the same patient (sometimes on the same day), then the number of times that the procedure was repeated is entered in the units field.
- *Exception:* If the procedure is an ASC procedure, the units field is not used to indicate that the procedure was performed more than once on the same day. The CPT code without the modifier 76 is reported to indicate the first time the procedure was performed. For each additional time the procedure was performed, repeat the CPT code with modifier 76 added.
- This modifier may be reported for services ordered by physicians but performed by technicians.

77   REPEAT PROCEDURE BY ANOTHER PHYSICIAN

The physician may need to indicate that a basic procedure or service performed by another physician had to be repeated. This situation may be reported by adding modifier 77 to the repeated procedure/service.

Coding Tips

- This modifier is used to indicate that a procedure performed by another physician had to be repeated in a separate operative session, on the same day.
- When the procedure is repeated on the same day but by another physician, the procedure code is reported once and then report it again with modifier 77 added (two line items).
- If the third-party payer requires a one line item only reporting of a procedure repeated on the same patient by a different physician (sometimes on the same day), then enter the number of times the procedure was repeated in the units field.
- *Exception:* If the procedure is an ASC procedure, the units field is not used to indicate that the procedure was performed more than once on the same day. The CPT code without the 77 modifier is reported to indicate the first time the procedure was performed and repeat the CPT code with modifier 77 added.
- This modifier may be reported for services ordered by physicians but performed by technicians.

✓ QUICK TIP

Hospital ASC and Outpatient Coders

Medicare's instructions for modifiers 76 and 77 in hospital ASC or hospital outpatient facilities include in the definition procedures "repeated in a separate operative session on the same calendar day." Use modifier 76 for same physician/same day and modifier 77 for another physician/same day. The procedure must be the same procedure.

78 RETURN TO THE OPERATING ROOM FOR A RELATED PROCEDURE DURING THE POSTOPERATIVE PERIOD

The physician may need to indicate that another procedure was performed during the postoperative period of the initial procedure. When this subsequent procedure is related to the first and requires the use of the operating room, it may be reported by adding the modifier 78 to the related procedure. (For repeat procedures on the same day, see modifier 76).

Coding Tips
- Consistent with the definition established by the AMA in CPT 2003, this modifier can be appended to the procedure code(s) when complications arise from the original surgery that require a return trip to the OR and/or when any related surgical procedures (that are not staged services) are performed in the OR.
- Do not report this modifier for procedures requiring a return to the OR that are repeat procedures or are unrelated to the original service(s) when performed by the same physician. (See modifiers 76 and 79, respectively, to report these circumstances with the appropriate modifier.)
- Reporting of this modifier may affect the adjudication process, causing the claim to be reviewed manually. Copies of medical record documentation may be requested to ensure the proper reporting of this modifier; therefore, documentation must firmly support the fact that a related procedure was performed during the postoperative period.

QUICK TIP

Hospital ASC and Outpatient Coders
Medicare's instructions for modifiers 78 and 79 in hospital ASC or hospital outpatient facilities include in the definition procedures "return to the operating room on the same day." Use modifier 78 for a procedure related to the initial procedure on the same day and modifier 79 for a procedure on the same day that is unrelated to the initial procedure.

79 UNRELATED PROCEDURE OR SERVICE BY THE SAME PHYSICIAN DURING THE POSTOPERATIVE PERIOD

The physician may need to indicate that the performance of a procedure or service during the postoperative period was unrelated to the original procedure. This circumstance may be reported by using modifier 79. (For repeat procedures on the same day, see modifier 76.)

Coding Tips
- Modifier 79 is reported to indicate that an unrelated procedure was performed by the same physician during the postoperative period of an original procedure or procedures.
- Do not report this modifier for procedures that are related to the original service(s). (See modifier 78 to report this circumstance.)
- Append this modifier to all unrelated procedures reported (not just on the first line-item) that are consistent with the definition of the modifier.

91 REPEAT CLINICAL DIAGNOSTIC LABORATORY TEST

In the course of treatment of the patient, it may be necessary to repeat the same laboratory test on the same day to obtain subsequent (multiple) test results. Under these circumstances, the laboratory test performed can be identified by its usual procedure number and the addition of modifier 91. **Note:** This modifier may not be used when tests are rerun to confirm initial results; due to testing problems with specimens or equipment; or for any other reason when a normal, one-time, reportable result is all that is required. This modifier may not be used when other code(s) describe a series of test results (e.g., glucose tolerance tests, evocative/

Ingenix Coding Lab: Understanding Modifiers

suppression testing). This modifier may only be used for laboratory test(s) performed more than once on the same day on the same patient.

Coding Tips

- Modifier 91 is added to the procedure code(s) that represent repeat laboratory tests or studies performed on the same day on the same patient.
- Add modifier 91 only when additional test results are to be obtained subsequent to the administration or performance of the same test(s) on the same day.
- Modifier 91 is not used when laboratory tests or studies are simply "rerun" because of specimen or equipment error or malfunction.
- Modifier 91 should not be reported when the basic procedure code(s) indicate that a series of test results are to be obtained, such as CPT code 82951 Glucose; tolerance test (GTT), three specimens (includes glucose).

HCPCS LEVEL II MODIFIERS

The following modifiers are available to report with CPT and HCPCS Level II codes for procedures performed on the eyelids, fingers, toes, specific sides of the body, a certain artery or for ambulance services. Using these modifiers prevents erroneous information from being reported with claim submissions.

The following modifiers are hospital-recognized modifiers (in alphabetical order):

E1   Upper left, eyelid

E2   Lower left, eyelid

E3   Upper right, eyelid

E4   Lower right, eyelid

FA   Left hand, thumb

F1   Left hand, second digit

F2   Left hand, third digit

F3   Left hand, fourth digit

F4   Left hand, fifth digit

F5   Right hand, thumb

F6   Right hand, second digit

F7   Right hand, third digit

F8   Right hand, fourth digit

F9   Right hand, fifth digit

GG   Performance and payment of a screening mammogram and diagnostic mammogram on the same patient, same day

GH   Diagnostic mammogram converted from screening mammogram on same day

---

✓ QUICK TIP

Referring physicians are required to provide diagnostic information to the testing entity at the time the test is ordered. All diagnostic tests must be ordered by the physician treating the beneficiary. An order may include the following forms of communication:

- A written document signed by the treating physician/practitioner, which is hand-delivered, mailed or faxed to the testing facility
- A telephone call by the treating physician/practitioner or his/her office to the testing facility
- An electronic mail by the treating physician/practitioner or his/her office to the testing facility

Note: If the order is communicated via telephone, both the treating physician/practitioner or his/her office and the testing facility must document the telephone call in their respective copies of the beneficiary's records.

©2003 Ingenix, Inc.
CPT only ©2003 American Medical Association. All Rights Reserved.

Chapter 8: ASC and Hospital Outpatient Modifiers

LC   Left circumflex coronary artery

- Use with codes 92980–92982, 92995 and 92996

LD   Left anterior descending coronary artery

- Use with codes 92980–92982, 92995 and 92996

LT   Left side

- Use to report procedures performed on the left side of the body.
- Do not use LT to report a bilateral surgical procedure.

QM   Ambulance service provided under arrangement by a provider of services

QN   Ambulance service furnished directly by a provider of services

RC   Right coronary artery

- Use with codes 92980–92982, 92995 and 92996

RT   Right side

- Use to report procedures performed on the right side of the body.
- Do not use RT to report a bilateral surgical procedure.

TA   Left foot, great toe

T1   Left foot, second digit

T2   Left foot, third digit

T3   Left foot, fourth digit

T4   Left foot, fifth digit

T5   Right foot, great toe

T6   Right foot, second digit

T7   Right foot, third digit

T8   Right foot, fourth digit

T9   Right foot, fifth digit

Note: HCPCS Level II modifiers recognized by the AMA and by CMS for hospital outpatient departments/clinics and ASCs may differ. It is highly recommended that each facility's coders check with the fiscal intermediary (FI) for Medicare claims, or check with the state Medicaid agency or various private payers to ascertain the appropriateness of assigning and subsequently reporting these special modifiers.

Additional HCPCS Level II modifiers may be necessary for reporting purposes, such as GH, diagnostic mammogram converted from screening mammogram on the same day; in these cases local FI policy may prevail.

©2003 Ingenix, Inc.

CPT only ©2003 American Medical Association. All Rights Reserved.

Chapter 9: Modifiers and Compliance

INTRODUCTION

Almost every segment of the health care industry has been affected by the federal government's antifraud and abuse campaigns over the last few years. Investigations of hospital billing practices, especially teaching hospitals, flooded the news media with reports of indictments, sanctions and out-of-court settlements for millions of dollars. With trepidation seeping into all areas of health care, more of the federal government's charges of fraud and abuse committed by clinical laboratories were heard nationwide, with tens of millions of dollars being paid back to the government. Home health agencies (HHAs), skilled nursing facilities, and durable medical equipment (DME) companies were then targeted. Finally, physician practices and ambulatory surgery centers (ASCs), in state after state, have been undergoing investigations by the FBI, the Office of the Inspector General (OIG), and by CMS officials. In June 2000, the OIG released a draft version of a physician compliance guidance document targeted to solo practitioners and small physician groups. The Federal Register of October 5, 2000, disclosed the final version of this compliance guidance. Given the fact that the federal government claims it has recouped inappropriate payments and overpayments and has collected fines totaling, up to this point, to several billion dollars, there are no signs that these fraud and abuse activities will wane.

This chapter of *Ingenix Coding Lab: Understanding Modifiers* explains the term "compliance" and provides an overview of the federal government's current efforts to eradicate fraud, waste, and abuse in health care programs. This chapter also provides the reader with logic trees for each modifier. The logic trees should be used by physicians and facilities as self-auditing tools to help ensure correct modifier usage.

WHAT IS COMPLIANCE?

Compliance is a broad term applied in recent years to certain aspects of the administrative side of health care. Compliance specifically encompasses the appropriate coding, billing (reporting), and documentation of medical services. In particular, being in compliance suggests the correct reporting of health care services to federal programs such as Medicare or the Children's Health Insurance Program (CHIP). This also applies to other federally funded programs, wholly or in part, such as state Medicaid or medical assistance programs. Under the Health Insurance Portability and Accountability Act (HIPAA) of 1996, even private payers have been empowered by this federal legislation to investigate, prosecute, and prevent health care fraud and abuse.

Most third-party payers, managed care organizations, preferred provider organizations, and the like have coding and billing guidelines that must be followed. Noncompliance or false reporting of services (fraud) can lead to expulsion from the

---

©2003 Ingenix, Inc.
CPT only ©2003 American Medical Association. All Rights Reserved.

plans, hefty penalties, and possible criminal charges. Expulsion from a major health care plan, such as Blue Shield, can permanently damage a medical practice's financial health. This is particularly true if the plan comprises a large percentage of the practice's patient base. Many of these payers will also publish the names and addresses of sanctioned providers, possibly leading to a marred reputation in the provider's professional community and difficulty in obtaining or retaining privileges at hospitals, nursing homes, etc.

Federal Fraud and Abuse Programs in Full Swing

The federal government's war on fraud and abuse has been very aggressive over the past several years, and continues to intensify. Spearheaded by the OIG of the Department of Health and Human Services (HHS), the FBI, the Department of Justice (DOJ) as well as CMS, the government has been very successful in uncovering more and more fraudulent activities aimed at the Medicare and Medicaid programs. These successful efforts have fueled and increased the intensity and number of investigations, and therefore there have been more indictments and convictions.

In recent years, a number of programs and initiatives have evolved out of HHS. All these parts together have come to form what HHS calls it's strategy to fight health care fraud, waste, and abuse. Parts of this strategy may already be familiar to physician office billers. A few of these programs and initiatives include:

Annual OIG Work Plan: In conjunction with CMS, the Public Health Service (PHS), and the Administrations for Children, Families, and Aging (all HHS entities), the OIG annual work plan mission statement reads, in part: "We improve HHS programs and operations, and protect them against fraud, waste and abuse. By conducting independent and objective audits, evaluations and investigations, we provide timely, useful and reliable information and advice to department officials, the administration, the Congress and the public." The OIG work plan assists the HHS in pursuing criminal convictions, by recovering maximum dollar amounts through judicial and administrative methods, and for recycling recouped program monies back into the federal programs.

Operation Restore Trust (ORT): This program was originally launched in five states to test several innovations in fighting Medicare and Medicaid fraud and abuse. It is now being expanded nationwide. ORT has been particularly adept at discovering Medicare overpayments to providers and hospitals.

Fraud and abuse hotline: HHS expanded the (800) HHS-TIPS hotline for reporting fraud in the Medicare and Medicaid programs. Since 1995, tips and complaints called into the program that have warranted specific follow-up action have numbered over 32,000.

Health Insurance Portability and Accountability Act (HIPAA): This 1996 law created a source of funding for HHS and DOJ to coordinate federal, state, and local health care law enforcement programs, conduct investigations, and provide guidance to the health care industry on fraudulent health care practices. It also established a national data bank to receive and report final adverse actions against unscrupulous health care providers and suppliers. With this increased funding the OIG now has offices operating in 38 states, and the Medicare program has increased claim reviews by 25 percent.

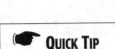

QUICK TIP

The "Silver" Army

Medicare patients signing up for combat? That's right…and they're turning out to be eager recruits, as well, in the government's campaign against health care fraud and abuse. The HHS in conjunction with the DOJ and the well-known third-party payer, the American Association of Retired Persons (AARP), have joined forces in a national effort called, "Who Pays? You Pay" to raise patient awareness of fraud and abuse within the Medicare program. Under the HHS, the three agencies involved in this front line effort are CMS, the OIG, and the Administration on Aging (AoA). Representatives from Medicare, the U.S. attorney general's office, the FBI, and the AARP are holding patient educational sessions in across the country, enlisting AoA senior Medicare patrol volunteers and AARP fraud fighters in this battle.

Medicare patients are being instructed to watch for and report the following activities:

- Duplicate billing of services
- Charges for services not performed or items not dispensed
- Inappropriate or unnecessary services
- Low-cost new or used medical equipment that is charged to the Medicare program as higher cost or new equipment
- Services free to the patient but billed to Medicare
- Certificates of medical necessity (CMNs) completed by the vendor instead of the provider

Chapter 9: Modifiers and Compliance

The Medical Integrity Program (MIP) and Payment Safeguards: This system of payment safeguards serves to identify and investigate suspicious claims throughout the Medicare program, and ensures that Medicare does not pay claims that other insurers should pay as the primary insurer. MIP also ensures that Medicare only pays for covered services that are reasonable and medically necessary. These safeguards attempt to identify improper claims before they are paid and prevent the need for Medicare to pay and chase.

Improving health care industry compliance: The OIG has issued compliance program guidance for clinical laboratories, hospitals, HHAs, third-party billing companies, and compliance guidance for the DMEPOS industry (including providers of DMEPOS and suppliers/vendors of DMEPOS). There is also a physician office compliance guidance document in the works.

Substantive claims testing: CMS is now working to develop a substantive testing process to help determine whether claims are paid properly, and also whether services are actually rendered and medically necessary.

Education efforts: CMS expects Medicare contractors to undertake educational efforts directed at the provider billing community about Medicare payment rules and fraudulent activity. This education will cover current payment policy, documentation requirements, and coding changes through quarterly bulletins, fraud alerts, and local seminars.

Budget year 2000 antifraud and abuse legislative package: President Clinton's FY 2000 budget proposal included further antifraud and antiabuse measures such as:

- Eliminating current requirements in federal law that require Medicare to make excessive payments for certain drugs; preventing abuse of Medicare's partial hospitalization benefit
- Ensuring that Medicare does not pay for claims liable to private insurers
- Expanding CMS contracting authority to purchase high-quality and cost-effective health care
- Expanding CMS's authority to terminate contractors who do not perform effectively.

Administration on Aging (AoA) fraud buster projects: The AoA is awarding $2 million in grants to 12 states to recruit and train thousands of retired professionals to serve as health care fraud busters who will work with older persons in their communities to review benefit statements and report potential cases of Medicare fraud, abuse, and program waste.

These programs, both singly and in combination, place a great deal of pressure on providers, coders, and billers to remain compliant with federal and state program directives and regulations. Consistent efforts in the areas of education; monitoring of documentation, coding, and billing practices; corrective action for uncovered errors or mistakes communicated by the Medicare and Medicaid programs; and prompt remittance of program overpayments have become absolutes in the physician and nonphysician practitioner billing realms. The health care industry buzz word compliance shows no signs of fading out.

QUICK TIP

In this era of increased federal investigations into physician and facility billing practices, it is prudent to conduct periodic internal audits. Doing so will help ensure billing compliance and accuracy in patient medical records. The following list details five areas of prevalent findings reported by federal or other third-party payer auditors after conducting on-site or off-site audits for HCPCS Level II coding and billing, including modifiers:

- Physician orders:
  - no physician orders on file
  - unsigned original orders
  - DMEPOS dispensed by not on orders
  - supplier forms not correlating to physician orders
  - diagnosis(ses) on claim not matching orders
  - orders unclear in directions/prescription
- Diagnosis coding:
  - truncated codes
  - wrong codes
  - claim, CMN or other forms/orders not reflective of assigned diagnosis(ses)
  - diagnosis does not support DMEPOS
- Service coding:
  - HCPCS code misrepresents the DMEPOS dispensed (upcoding [e.g. coding a splint as a brace or orthotic])
  - unlisted HCPCS code used when a listed code exists
  - code (service) not supported by diagnosis(ses)
  - wrong HCPCS Level II code
  - HCPCS Level II modifier not applicable with HCPCS Level II code reported
  - HCPCS Level II modifier not applicable with CPT code reported
  - missing HCPCS Level II modifier(s)
- Medical records:
  - date of service not entered
  - mismatching dates of service (forms do not match record)
  - incomplete data in record
  - diagnosis(ses) not found in chart under date of service specified
  - chart not located
  - notes illegible
- Claims:
  - misslinked service and diagnosis codes
  - unlinked service and diagnosis codes
  - unlisted HCPCS codes without explanation
  - use of 99070 on DMERC claims
  - claims filed to wrong entity
  - UPIN not noted for referring physician
  - wrong HIC number for patient*

©2003 Ingenix, Inc.
CPT only ©2003 American Medical Association. All Rights Reserved.

The OIG's Compliance Plan Guidance

The *Federal Register* of October 5, 2000, contained the federal government's final version of the OIG's Compliance Program for Individual and Small Group Physician Practices. At an earlier press conference for the release of this plan, OIG representatives stated that "this voluntary compliance guidance should assist providers in preventing the submission of erroneous claims or in engaging in unlawful conduct for federal health care programs." While the specifics of this compliance guidance document are beyond the scope of this publication, the basic tenets of all of the OIG's compliance guidance documents are reiterated in the compliance guidance for physicians. These tenets include:

- Development and distribution of written standards of conduct, as well as written policies and procedures, which promote the provideri's commitment to compliance (e.g., by including adherence to the compliance program as an element in evaluating managers and employees), and which must also address specific areas of potential fraud, such as claims development and submission processes
- Designation of a compliance officer and other appropriate bodies (e.g., a corporate compliance committee) charged with the responsibility for operating and monitoring the compliance program, and who report directly to the CEO and/ or the governing body It is important that the compliance program is structured in such a way to allow the compliance officials to accomplish the key functions of the compliance plan without interference from middle managers, practice administrators, and financial officers other than the CEO and/or governing body
- Development and implementation of consistent and effective education and training programs for pertinent employees. These training and education programs should be detailed and comprehensive. They should cover specific coding and billing procedures, including the application of modifiers, and areas of concern in medical record documentation. For DMEPOS suppliers, the sales and marketing practices of the company should be addressed
- Development of effective lines of communication, such as the creation and maintenance of a hotline or other reporting mechanism to receive fraud and abuse complaints. In this process, the adoption of procedures to protect the anonymity of complainants and procedures to protect callers/employees from retaliation should likewise be developed
- Development of a system to respond to allegations of improper/illegal activities and the enforcement of appropriate disciplinary action against employees who have violated internal compliance policies, applicable statutes, regulations, or federal, state, and private payer health care program requirements. The development of a policy (or policies) that addresses the parameters for retention of sanctioned individuals is also a critical aspect of this element of an effective compliance plan
- Use of audits and/or other risk evaluation techniques to regularly monitor compliance, identify problem areas, and assist in the reduction of identified problem areas. For example, the periodic spot-checking the work of coding and billing personnel should be an element of an effective compliance program
- Prompt response to detected offenses and the development of corrective action plans, when necessary. The investigation and corrective action of identified problems must be an active element in the compliance program.

☞ Quick Tip

If a third-party billing company discovers credible evidence of a provider's misconduct, or flagrant fraudulent or abusive conduct, the company should:

- Refrain from submitting any false or inappropriate claims
- Notify the provider of the findings
- Request corrected information for claim resubmission
- Terminate the contract if the provider does not respond to inquiries
- Report the misconduct, and if the provider does not take corrective action, to the appropriate federal and state authorities within a reasonable time frame (i.e., no more than 60 days after determining that there is credible evidence of a violation)

Benefits of a Compliance Program

According to the OIG, an effective compliance program provides a mechanism that brings the public and private sectors together to reach mutual goals of reducing fraud and abuse, improving operational quality, improving the quality of health care services and ultimately reducing the cost of health care. In addition to fulfilling its legal duty to ensure that it is not submitting false or inaccurate claims to governmental and private payers, providers and suppliers may gain numerous additional benefits by voluntarily implementing an effective compliance program. These benefits may include the following:

- The formulation of effective internal controls to ensure compliance with federal and state statutes, rules, and regulations, and federal, state, and private payer health care program requirements and internal guidelines
- A concrete demonstration to employees and the community at large of the provider's strong commitment to honest and responsible conduct
- The ability to obtain an accurate assessment of employee and contractor behavior relating to fraud and abuse
- An increased likelihood of identification and prevention of criminal and unethical conduct
- The ability to more quickly and accurately react to employee operational compliance concerns and the capability to effectively target resources to address those concerns
- Improvement of the quality, efficiency, and consistency of providing services

Increased employee efficiency:

- A centralized source for distributing information on health care statutes, regulations, policies, and other program directives regarding fraud and abuse issues

Improved internal communication:

- A methodology that encourages employees to report potential problems
- Procedures that allow the prompt, thorough investigation of alleged misconduct by corporate officers, managers, sales representatives, employees, independent contractors, consultants, clinicians, and other health care professionals
- Initiation of immediate, appropriate, and decisive corrective action
- Early detection and reporting, minimizing the loss to the government from false claims, and thereby reducing the provider's exposure to civil damages and penalties, criminal sanctions, and administrative remedies, such as program exclusion.

Implementation of a compliance program may allow federal auditors to recognize the fact that the provider or supplier instituted a compliance program that predates a federal or state investigation; this in turn may have influence over the assessment of sanctions. However, the burden is on the provider to demonstrate the operational effectiveness of the compliance program. Overall, the OIG believes that an effective compliance program is a sound investment on the part of a health care provider as it can significantly reduce the risk of unlawful or improper conduct.

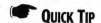

QUICK TIP

DMEPOS Industry Is Given Guidelines for Compliance

The durable medical equipment, prosthetics, orthotics and supplies (DMEPOS) industry sat up and took notice of the much anticipated OIG's compliance program for providers and suppliers of DMEPOS items and services. The voluntary program is similar to the other compliance programs released by the OIG for clinical laboratories, hospitals, HHAs, and third-party medical billing companies. The DMEPOS compliance program is designed to assist in the elimination of fraud and abuse within the DMEPOS provider/supplier industry.

MODIFIERS AND COMPLIANCE: A QUICK SELF-TEST

A cardiology practice in the Midwest was audited and fined by the federal government for inaccurate coding and lack of medical record documentation. An ophthalmology practice located in the Northwest underwent an audit by a state Medicaid program and was found to have duplicate billings, unbundling of services, and inappropriate use of ophthalmological codes. A multispecialty practice in the West succumbed to federal auditors and was charged with abusive billing practices, which included the inappropriate use of modifiers.

With federal and state activities to uncover health care fraud and abuse reaching a fever pitch, many physician offices and billing services have begun to implement internal controls to ensure appropriate billing practices, including internal investigations of the use of modifiers. Here's a quick checklist for your practice to follow in this endeavor. It's not all-inclusive, but it can help you remain compliant when reporting modifiers.

An answer of yes to the following questions is essential for fraud and abuse compliance:

- Do you carefully review all pertinent documentation prior to appending a CPT or HCPCS Level II code with a modifier?
- Do you monitor the activities of your billing office or service with respect to modifier usage (e.g., are you notified of denials and requests for more information) and if you use a billing service are you furnished with monthly reports that detail all claims submitted?
- Do you randomly cross-check all billings performed by your billing office or service to be certain that all claims submitted with modifiers are accurate, and is each modifier reported appropriate to the clinical situation or circumstance noted in the patientís chart?
- Do you hold inservice educational sessions on Medicare and Medicaid program changes in modifier reporting, as well as other coding, billing, and documentation requirements?
- Are all of the services billed to Medicare and Medicaid thoroughly documented in the patients' medical records?
- Are new billing employees immediately oriented in the modifier reporting policies and procedures for both Medicare and Medicaid? Other major third-party payers?

An answer of no to the following questions is essential for fraud and abuse compliance:

- Do you allow your billing office or service to assign modifiers and subsequently report services on claims without conducting an intermittent (or regularly scheduled) review of claims, including electronic submissions?
- Does your billing office or service have carte blanche permission to correct and/ or change codes (CPT, ICD-9-CM, HCPCS Level II, and modifiers) for services that you have performed?
- Is there evidence of inappropriate overpayment by the payer when a modifier is used?
- Does your billing office or service answer all Medicare and Medicaid inquiries regarding your services and claims on your behalf, without your knowledge?

©2003 Ingenix, Inc.

CPT only ©2003 American Medical Association. All Rights Reserved.

- Do you refrain from sending your billing staff to educational seminars because you feel that this is not necessary?
- Do you allow new billing employees to sign claims on your behalf?
- Do Medicare and other payers repeatedly seem to disregard your modifier reporting (i.e., there are no adjustments made to the typical reimbursements for services billed with modifiers) or, are your claims repeatedly denied when submitted with modifiers? (An answer of no may suggest inappropriate application of modifiers and/or lack of understanding of modifier definitions and use.)

On the following pages are flow charts coders can follow when deciding on which modifier to use and whether additional documentation might be required.

Ingenix Coding Lab: Understanding Modifiers

Modifier 21

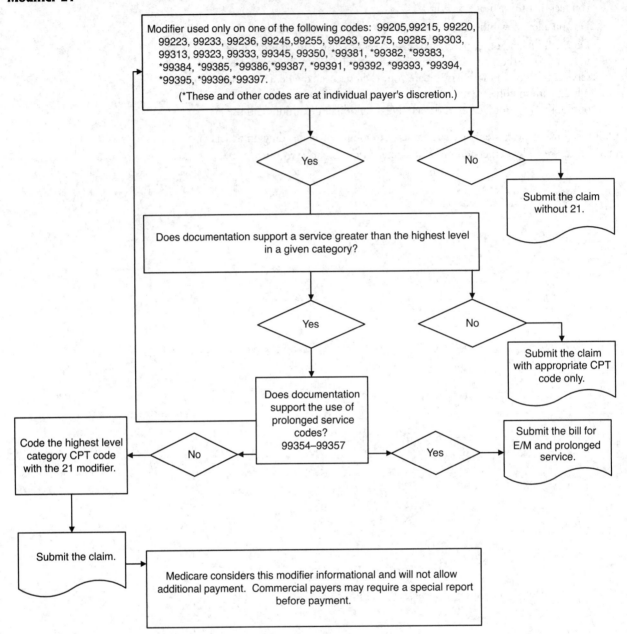

Chapter 9: Modifiers and Compliance

Modifier 22

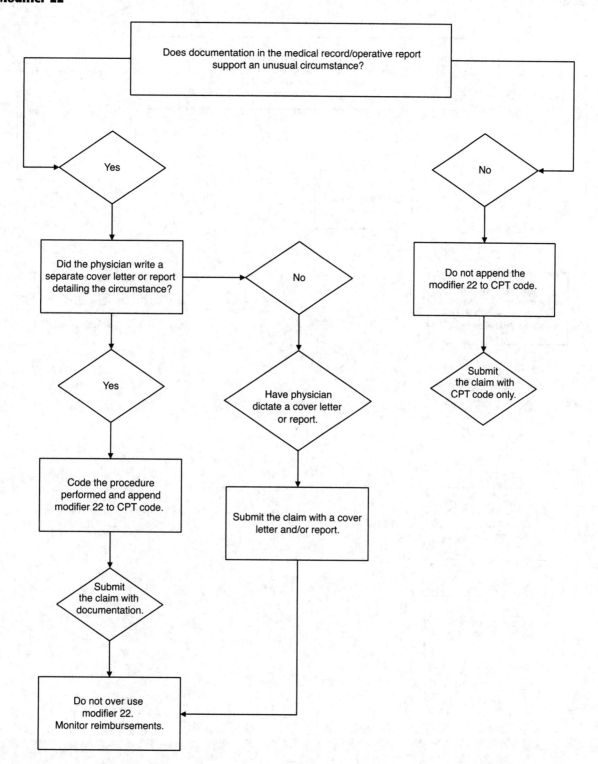

Ingenix Coding Lab: Understanding Modifiers

Modifier 23

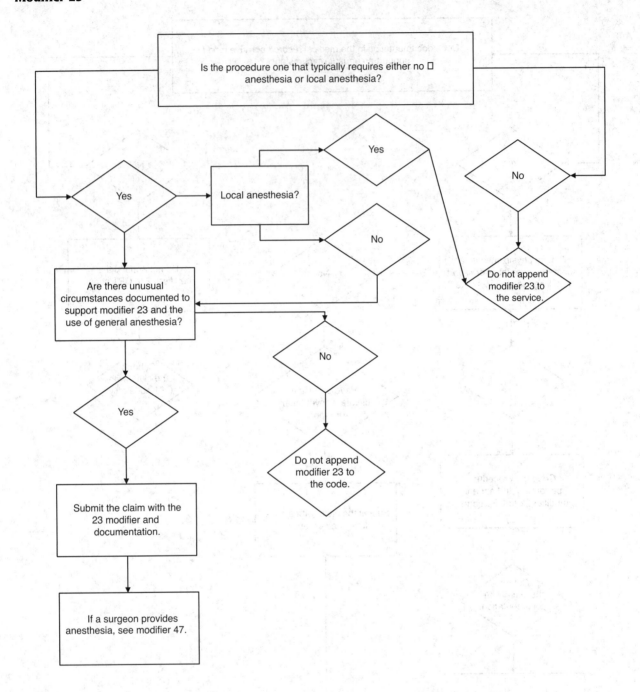

Modifier 24

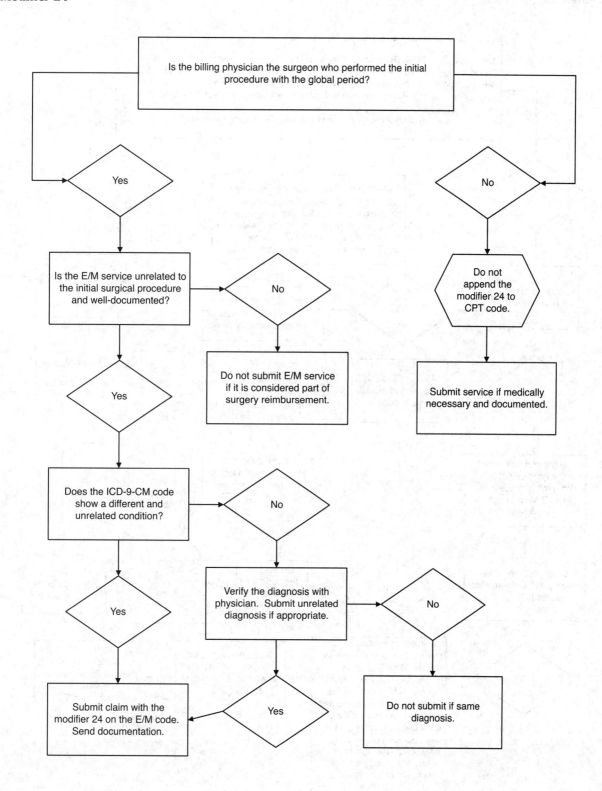

Ingenix Coding Lab: Understanding Modifiers

Modifier 25

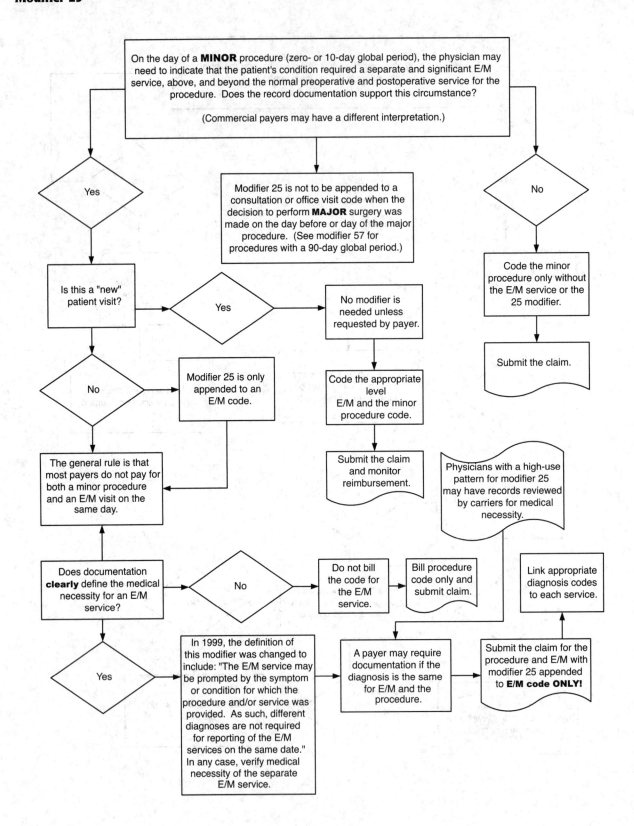

Chapter 9: Modifiers and Compliance

Modifier 26

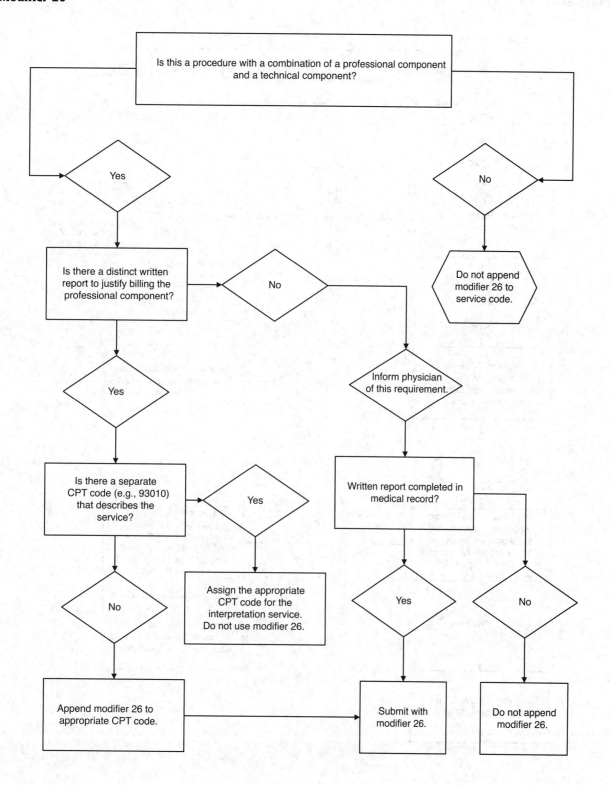

Ingenix Coding Lab: Understanding Modifiers

Modifier 27

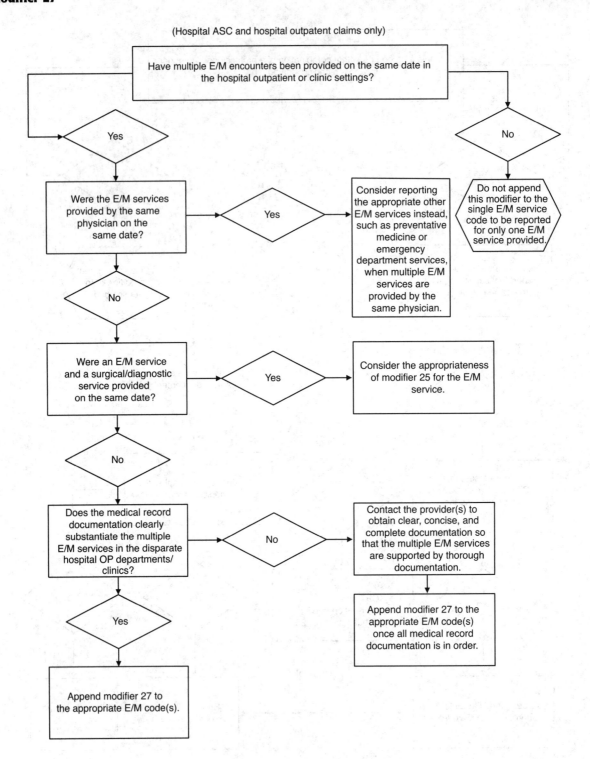

Chapter 9: Modifiers and Compliance

Modifier 32

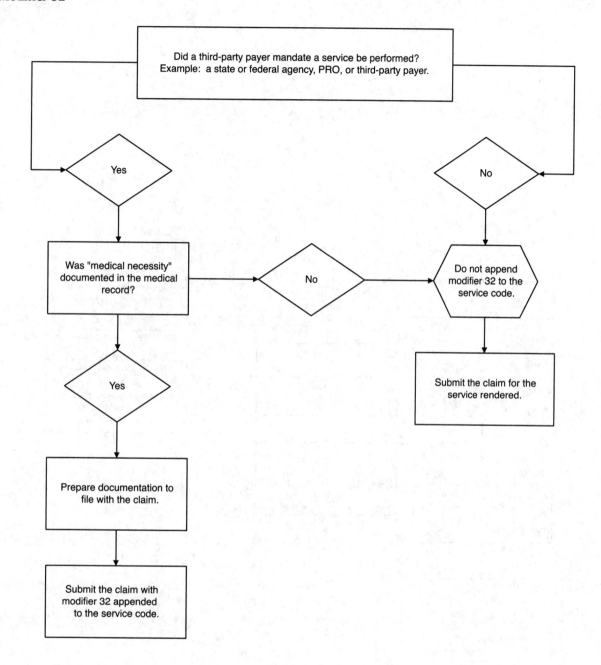

Ingenix Coding Lab: Understanding Modifiers

Modifier 47

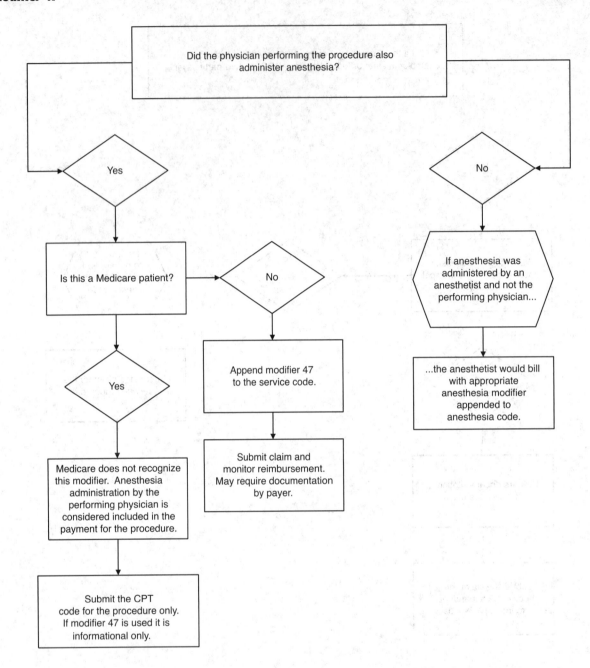

Chapter 9: Modifiers and Compliance

Modifier 50

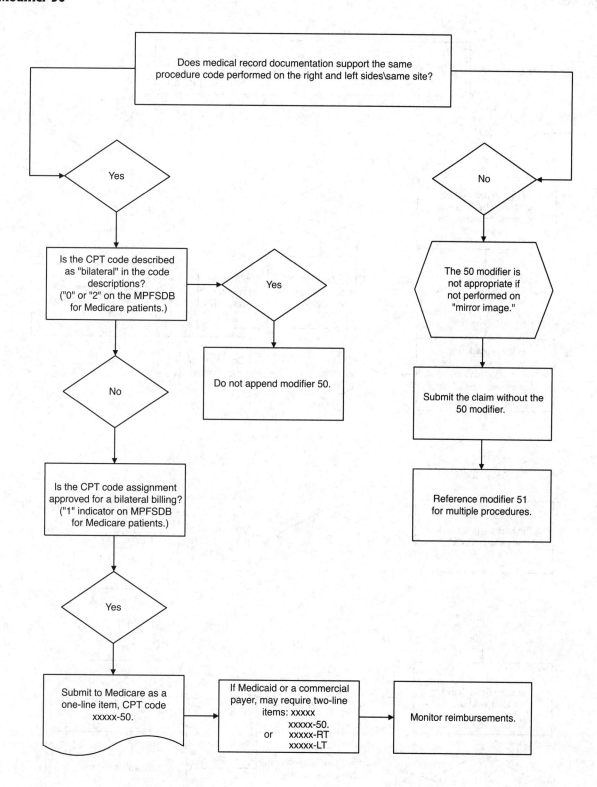

Ingenix Coding Lab: Understanding Modifiers

Modifier 51

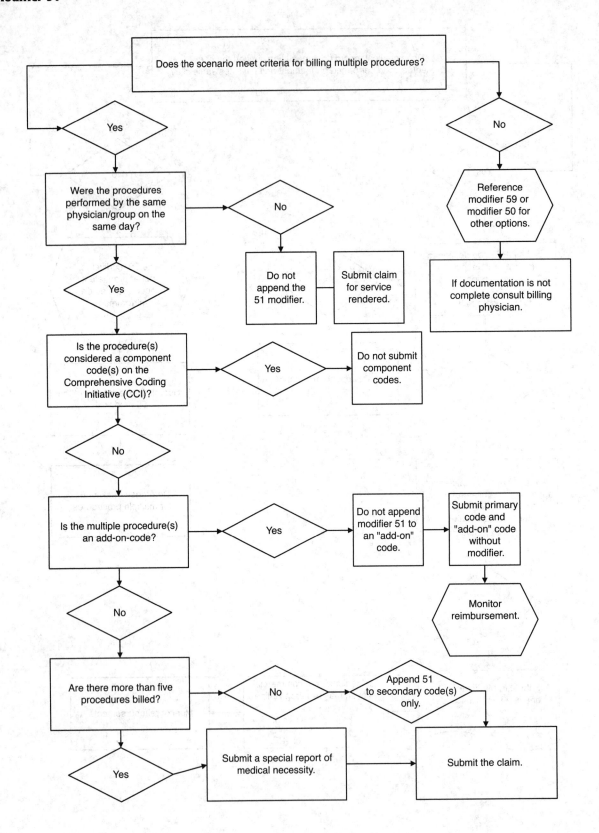

Chapter 9: Modifiers and Compliance

Modifier 52

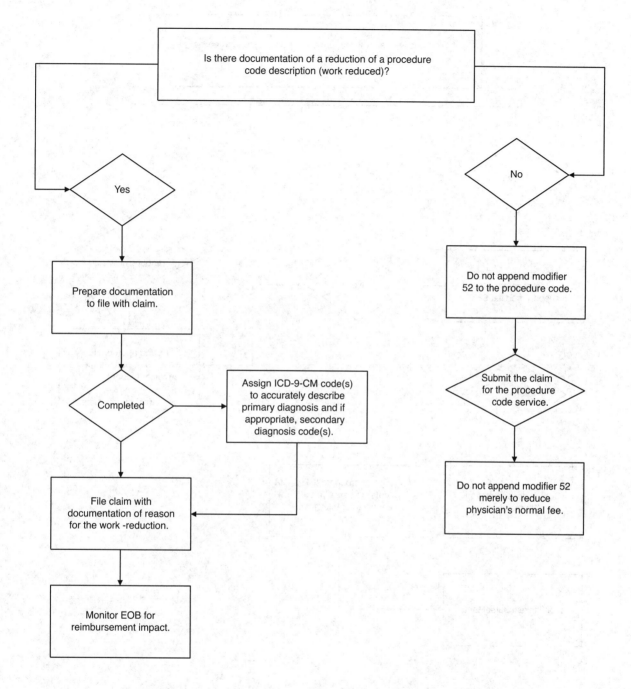

Per Medicare, modifier 52, Reduced service, is used in the hospital outpatient department to identify a procedure not requiring anesthesia (meaning general, regional, or local) that was terminated after the patient was prepared for the procedure (including any sedation). Reimbursement for modifier 52 procedures is 50 percent.

©2003 Ingenix, Inc.
CPT only ©2003 American Medical Association. All Rights Reserved.

165

Modifier 53

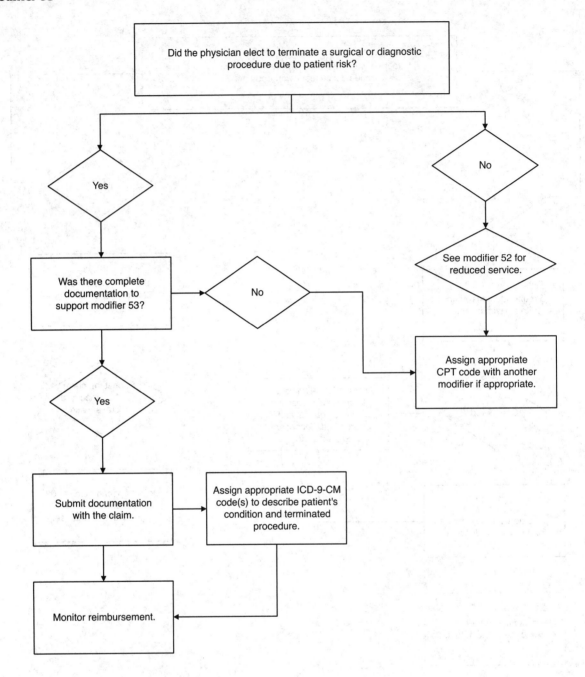

Chapter 9: Modifiers and Compliance

Modifier 54

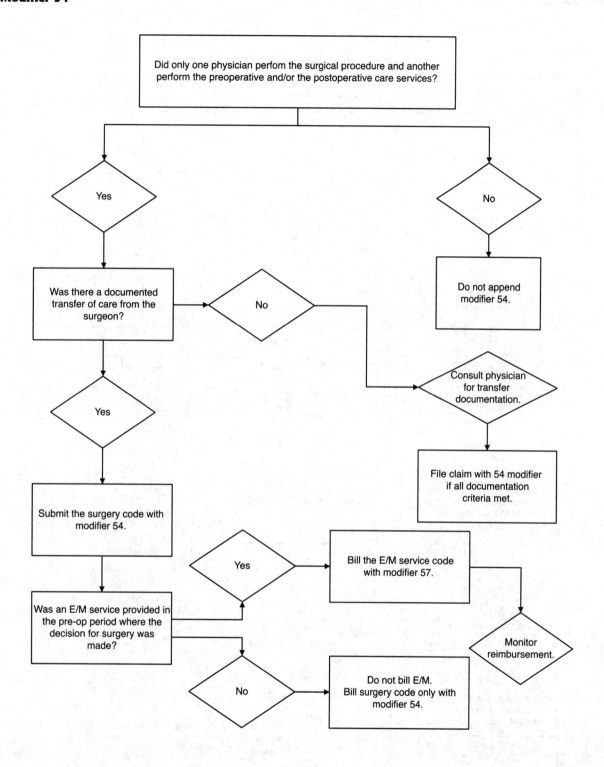

Modifier 55

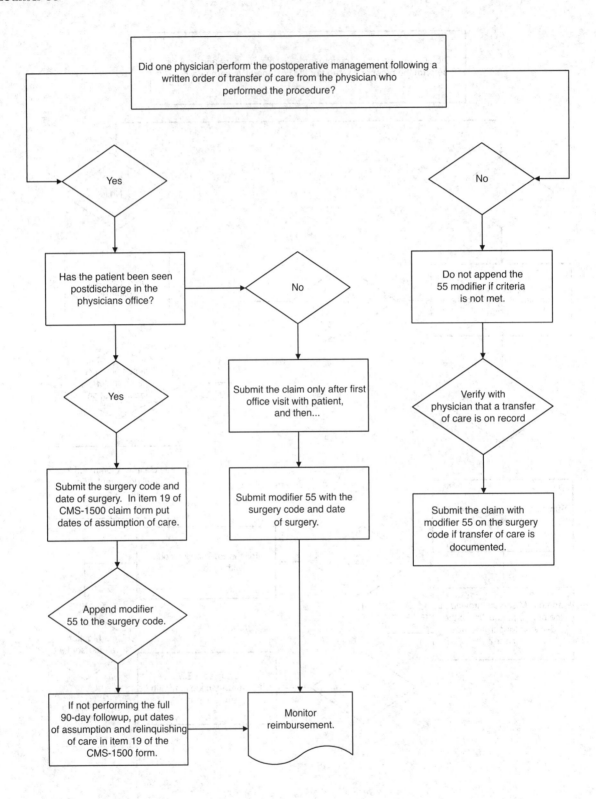

Modifier 56

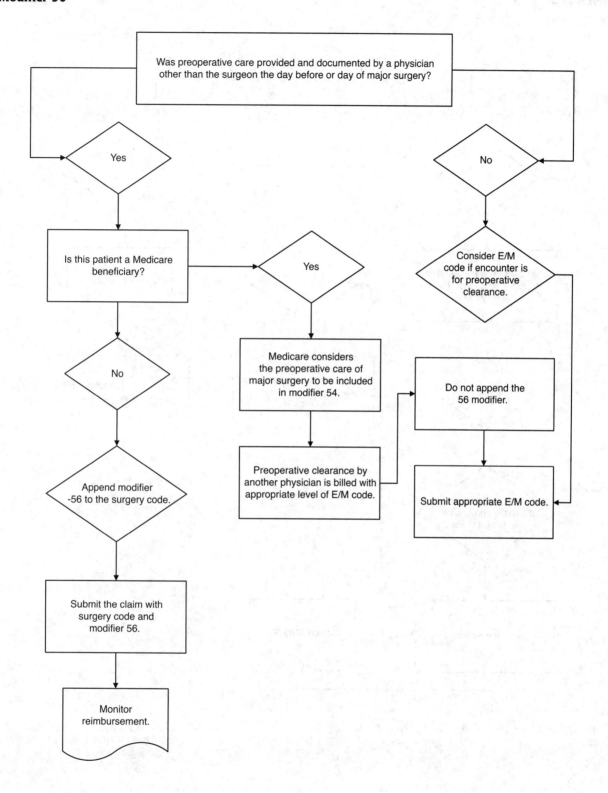

Ingenix Coding Lab: Understanding Modifiers

Modifier 57

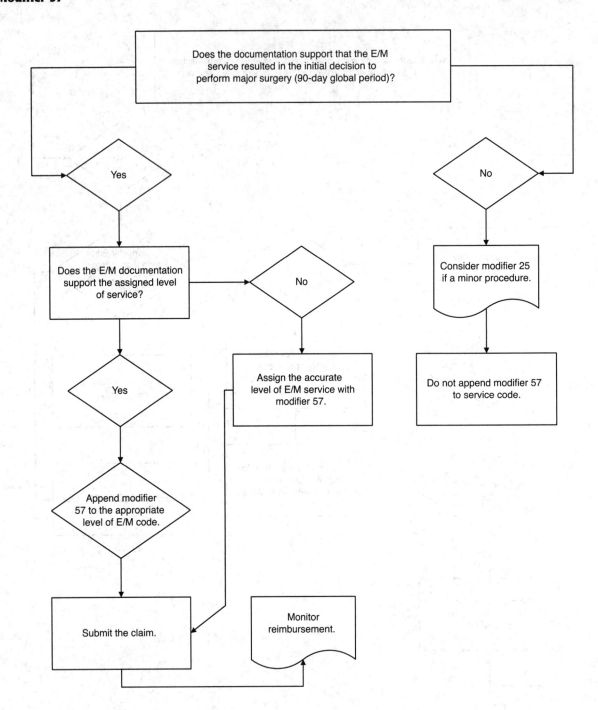

Chapter 9: Modifiers and Compliance

Modifier 58

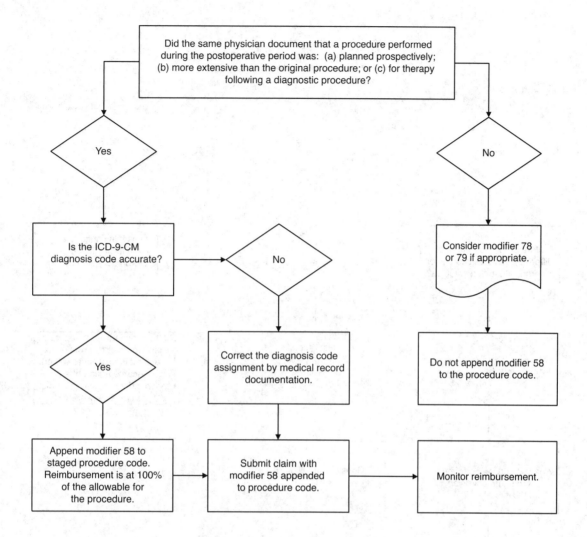

Note: Postoperative period for Hospital Outpatient Prospective Payment Claims is defined as same calendar day.

Ingenix Coding Lab: Understanding Modifiers

Modifier 59

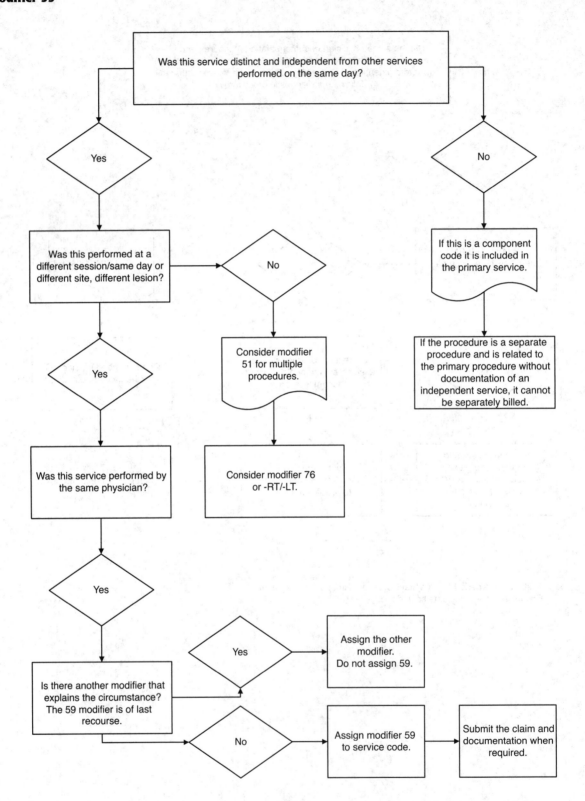

Chapter 9: Modifiers and Compliance

Modifier 62

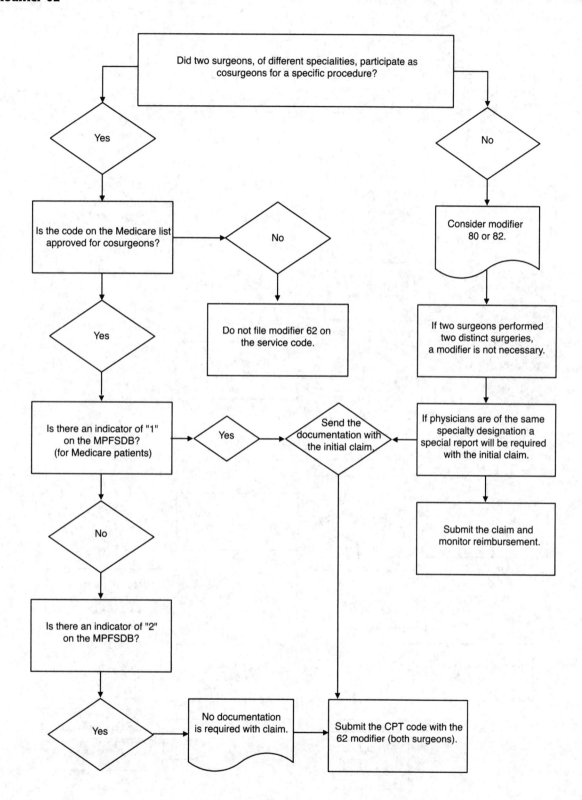

Ingenix Coding Lab: Understanding Modifiers

Modifier 63

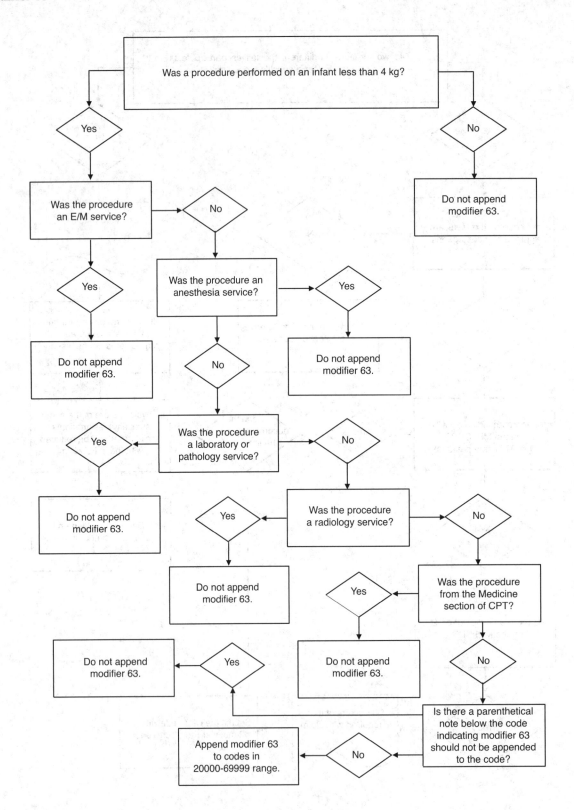

Modifier 66

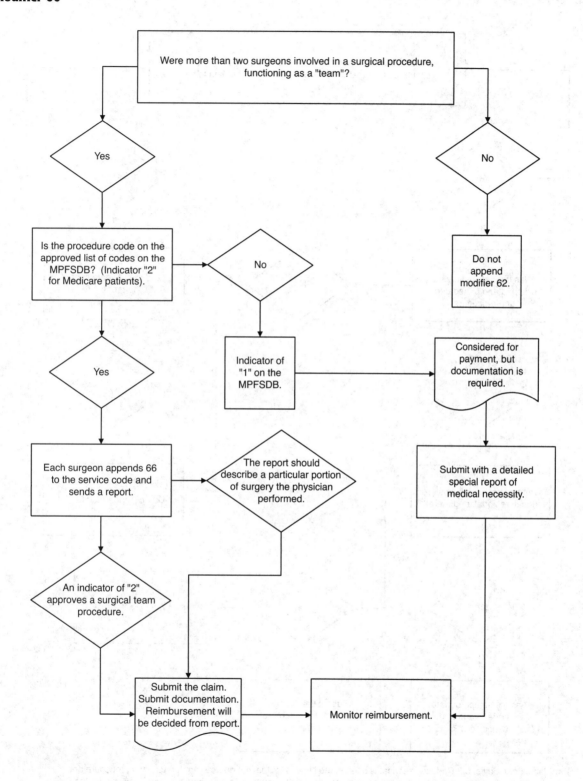

Ingenix Coding Lab: Understanding Modifiers

Modifier 73

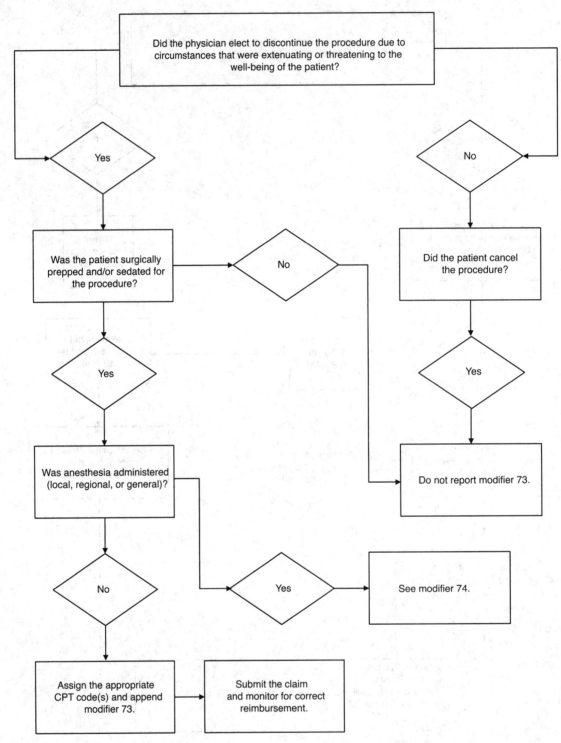

Per Medicare, modifier 52, Reduced service, is used in the hospital outpatient department to identify a procedure not requiring anesthesia (meaning general, regional, or local) that was terminated after the patient was prepared for the procedure (including any sedation). Reimbursement for modifier 52 procedures is 50 percent.

Ingenix Coding Lab: Understanding Modifiers

Modifier 74

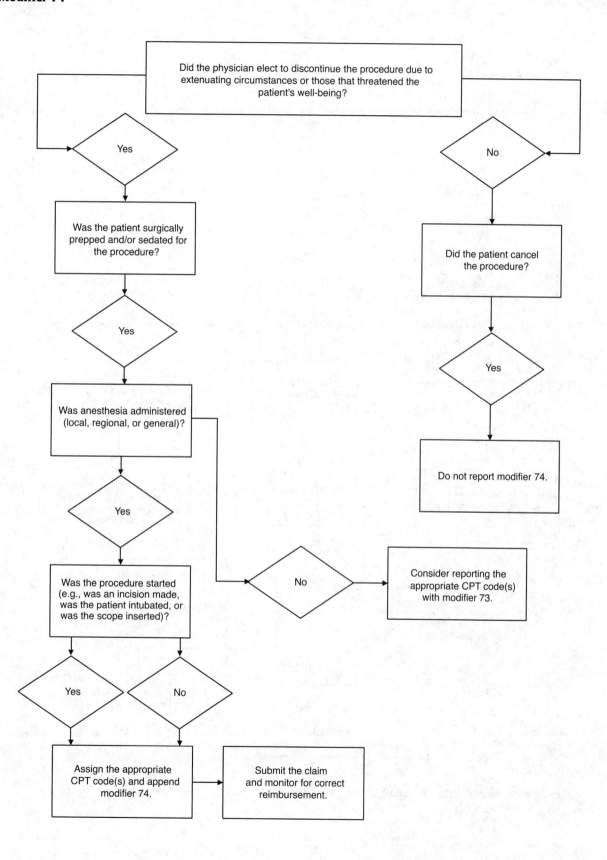

Ingenix Coding Lab: Understanding Modifiers

Modifier 76

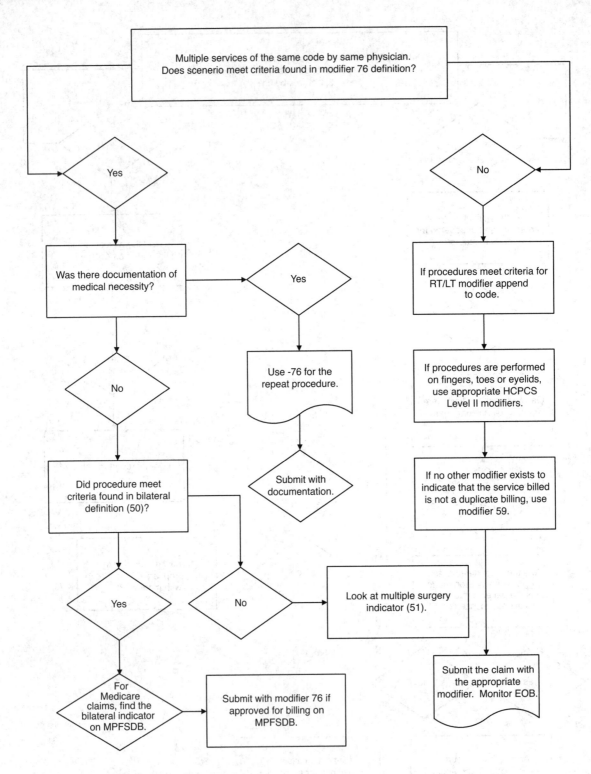

Note: Postoperative period for Hospital Outpatient Prospective Payment Claims is defined as same calendar day.

Chapter 9: Modifiers and Compliance

Modifier 77

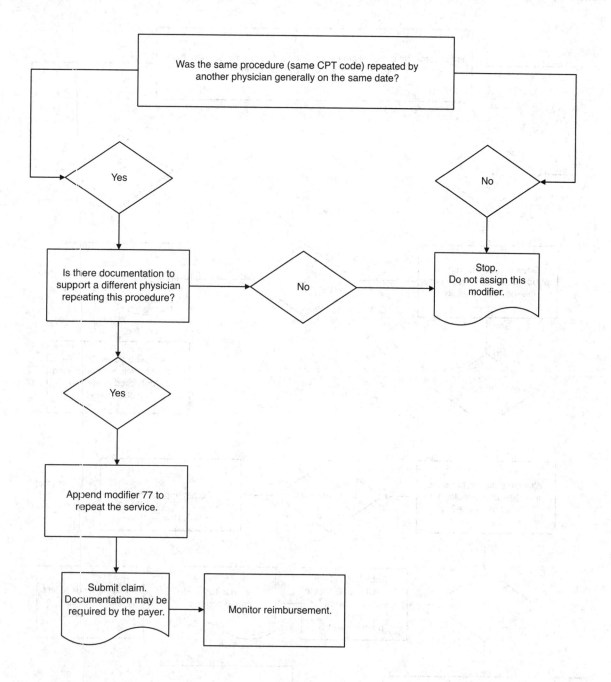

Note: Postoperative period for Hospital Outpatient Prospective Payment claims is defined as same calendar day.

Ingenix Coding Lab: Understanding Modifiers

Modifier 78

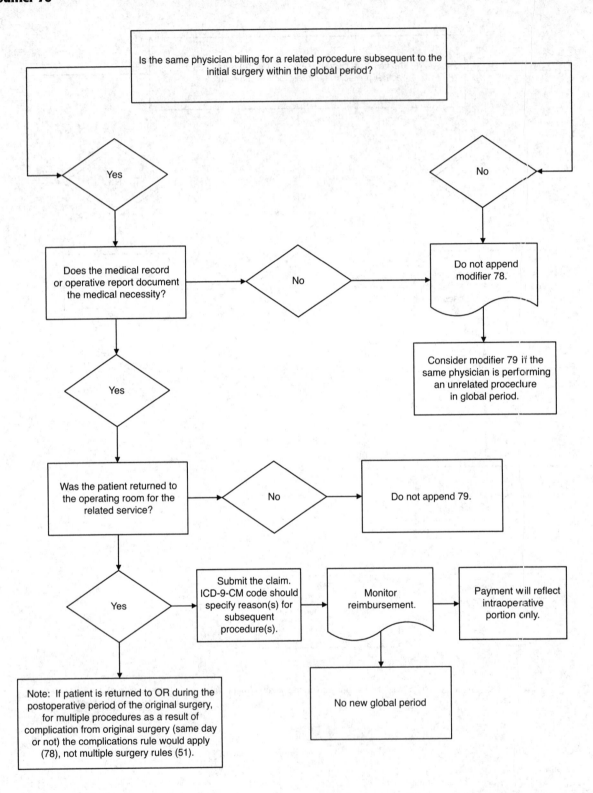

Note: Postoperative period for Hospital Outpatient Prospective Payment claims is defined as same calendar day.

Modifier 79

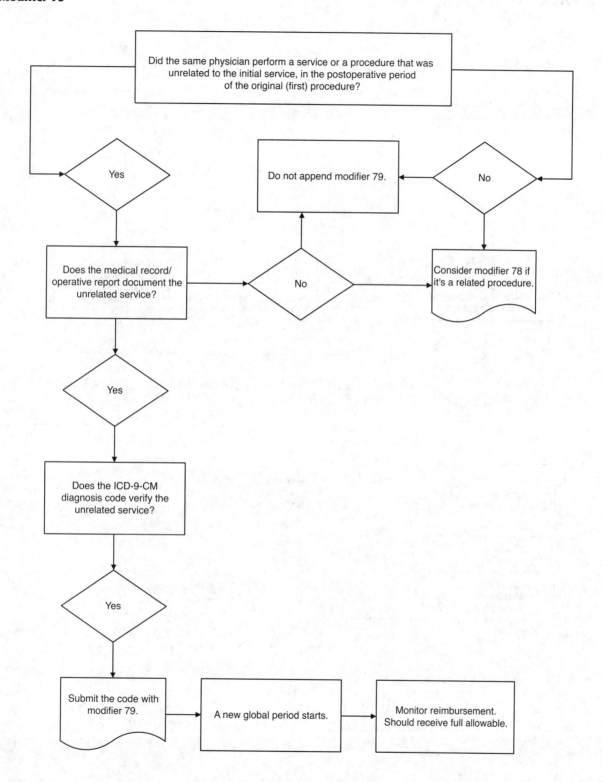

Note: Postoperative period for Hospital Outpatient Prospective Payment claims is defined as same calendar day.

Ingenix Coding Lab: Understanding Modifiers

Modifier 80

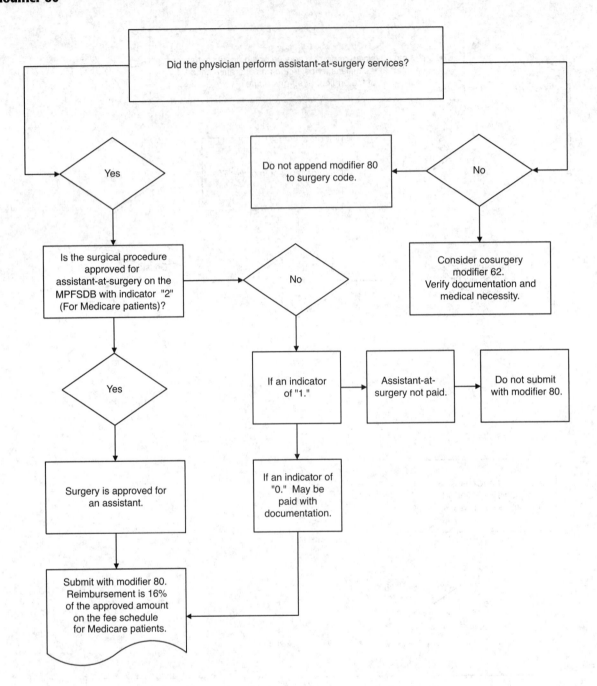

Modifier 81

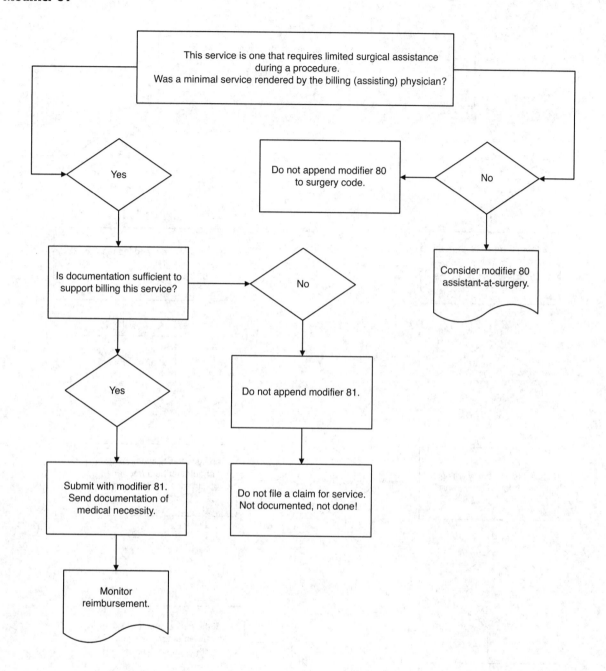

Ingenix Coding Lab: Understanding Modifiers

Modifier 82

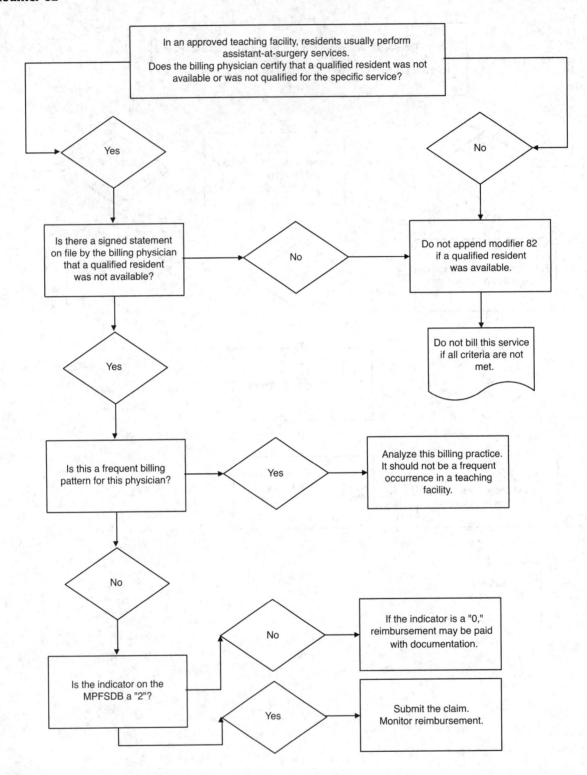

Modifier 90

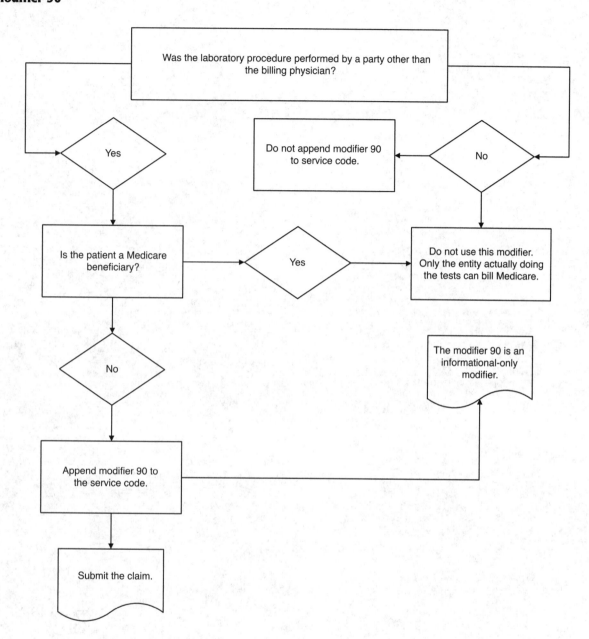

Chapter 10: Modifier Descriptors

21   **Prolonged evaluation and management services:** When the face-to-face or floor/unit service(s) provided is prolonged or otherwise greater than that usually required for the highest level of evaluation and management service within a given category, it may be identified by adding modifier 21 to the evaluation and management code number. A report may also be appropriate.

22   **Unusual procedural services:** When the service(s) provided is greater than that usually required for the listed procedure, it may be identified by adding modifier 22 to the usual procedure number. A report may also be appropriate.

23   **Unusual anesthesia:** Occasionally, a procedure, which usually requires either no anesthesia or local anesthesia, because of unusual circumstances must be done under general anesthesia. This circumstance may be reported by adding the modifier 23 to the procedure code of the basic service.

24   **Unrelated evaluation and management service by the same physician during a postoperative period:** The physician may need to indicate that an evaluation and management service was performed during a postoperative period for a reason(s) unrelated to the original procedure. This circumstance may be reported by adding the modifier 24 to the appropriate level of E/M service.

25   **Significant, separately identifiable evaluation and management service by the same physician on the same day of the procedure or other service:** The physician may need to indicate that on the day a procedure or service identified by a CPT code was performed, the patient's condition required a significant, separately identifiable E/M service above and beyond the other service provided or beyond the usual preoperative and postoperative care associated with the procedure that was performed. The E/M service may be prompted by the symptom or condition for which the procedure and/or service was provided. As such, different diagnoses are not required for reporting of the E/M services on the same date. This circumstance may be reported by adding the modifier 25 to the appropriate level of E/M service. **Note:** This modifier is not used to report an E/M service that resulted in a decision to perform surgery. See modifier 57.

26   **Professional component:** Certain procedures are a combination of a physician component and a technical component. When the physician component is reported separately, the service may be identified by adding the modifier 26 to the usual procedure number.

©2003 Ingenix, Inc.
CPT only ©2003 American Medical Association. All Rights Reserved.

27 **Multiple outpatient hospital E/M encounters on the same date:** For hospital outpatient reporting purposes, utilization of hospital resources related to separate and distinct E/M encounters performed in multiple outpatient hospital settings on the same date may be reported by adding the modifier 27 to each appropriate level outpatient and/or emergency department (E/M) code(s). This modifier provides a means of reporting circumstances involving management services provided by physician(s) in more than one (multiple) outpatient hospital setting(s) (e.g., hospital emergency department, clinic). **Note:** This modifier is not to be used for physician reporting of multiple E/M services performed by the same physician on the same date. For physician reporting of all outpatient E/M services provided by the same physician on the same date and performed in multiple outpatient setting(s) (e.g., hospital emergency department, clinic), see evaluation and management, emergency department, or preventive medicine services codes.

32 **Mandated services:** Services related to mandated consultation and/or related services (e.g., PRO, third-party payer, governmental, legislative, or regulatory requirement) may be identified by adding the modifier 32 to the basic procedure.

47 **Anesthesia by surgeon:** Regional or general anesthesia provided by the surgeon may be reported by adding the modifier 47 to the basic service. (This does not include local anesthesia.) **Note:** Modifier 47 would not be used as a modifier for the anesthesia procedures 00100–01999.

50 **Bilateral procedure:** Unless otherwise identified in the listings, bilateral procedures that are performed at the same operative session should be identified by adding the modifier 50 to the appropriate five-digit code.

51 **Multiple procedures:** When multiple procedures, other than evaluation and management services, are performed at the same session by the same provider, the primary procedure or service may be reported as listed. The additional procedure(s) or service(s) may be identified by appending the modifier 51 to the additional procedure or service code(s). **Note:** This modifier should not be appended to designated add-on codes.

52 **Reduced services:** Under certain circumstances a service or procedure is partially reduced or eliminated at the physician's discretion. Under these circumstances the service provided can be identified by its usual procedure number and the addition of the modifier 52, signifying that the service is reduced. This provides a means of reporting reduced services without disturbing the identification of the basic service. **Note:** For hospital outpatient reporting of a previously scheduled procedure/service that is partially reduced or canceled as a result of extenuating circumstances or those that threaten the well-being of the patient prior to or after administration of anesthesia, see modifiers 73 and 74.

53 **Discontinued procedure:** Under certain circumstances, the physician may elect to terminate a surgical or diagnostic procedure. Due to extenuating circumstances or those that threaten the well-being of the patient, it may be necessary to indicate that a surgical or diagnostic procedure was started but discontinued. This circumstance may be reported by adding the modifier 53 to the code reported by the physician for the discontinued procedure. **Note:** This modifier is not used to report the elective cancellation of a procedure prior to the patient's anesthesia induction and/or surgical preparation in the operating suite. For outpatient hospital/ambulatory surgery center (ASC) reporting of a previously scheduled procedure/service that is partially reduced or canceled as a result of extenuating circumstances or those that threaten the well-being of the patient prior to or after administration of anesthesia, see modifiers 73 and 74.

54 **Surgical care only:** When one physician performs a surgical procedure and another provides preoperative and/or postoperative management, surgical services may be identified by adding the modifier 54 to the usual procedure number.

55 **Postoperative management only:** When one physician performs the postoperative management and another physician has performed the surgical procedure, the postoperative component may be identified by adding the modifier 55 to the usual procedure number.

56 **Preoperative management only:** When one physician performs the preoperative care and evaluation and another physician performs the surgical procedure, the preoperative component may be identified by adding the modifier 56 to the usual procedure number.

57 **Decision for surgery:** An E/M service that resulted in the initial decision to perform the surgery may be identified by adding the modifier 57 to the appropriate level of E/M service.

58 **Staged or related procedure or service by the same physician during the postoperative period:** The physician may need to indicate that the performance of a procedure or service during the postoperative period was: a) planned prospectively at the time of the original procedure (staged); b) more extensive than the original procedure; or c) for therapy following a diagnostic surgical procedure. This circumstance may be reported by adding the modifier 58 to the staged or related procedure. **Note:** this modifier is not used to report the treatment of a problem that requires a return to the operating room. See modifier 78.

59 **Distinct procedural service:** Under certain circumstances, the physician may need to indicate that a procedure or service was distinct or independent from other services performed on the same day. Modifier 59 is used to identify procedures/services that are not normally reported together but are appropriate under the circumstances. This may represent a different session or patient encounter, different procedure or surgery, different site or organ system, separate incision/excision, separate lesion, or separate injury (or area of injury in extensive injuries) not ordinarily encountered or performed on the same day by the same physician. However, when another already established modifier is appropriate it should be used rather than modifier 59. Only if no more descriptive modifier is available, and the use of modifier 59 best explains the circumstances, should modifier 59 be used.

©2003 Ingenix, Inc.
CPT only ©2003 American Medical Association. All Rights Reserved.

62	**Two surgeons:** When two surgeons work together as primary surgeons performing distinct part(s) of a procedure, each surgeon should report his/her distinct operative work by adding modifier 62 to the procedure code and any associated add-on code(s) for that procedure as long as both surgeons continue to work together as primary surgeons. Each surgeon should report the cosurgery once using the same procedure code. If additional procedure(s) (including add-on procedure[s]) are performed during the same surgical session, separate code(s) may also be reported with modifier 62. **Note:** If a cosurgeon acts as an assistant in the performance of additional procedure(s) during the same surgical session, those services may be reported using separate procedure code(s) with modifier 80 or modifier 82 added, as appropriate.
63	**Procedure performed on infants less than 4 kg:** Procedures performed on neonates and infants up to a present body weight of 4 kg may involve significantly increased complexity and physician work commonly associated with these patients. This circumstance may be reported by adding the modifier 63 to the procedure number. **Note:** Unless otherwise designated, this modifier may be appended only to the procedures/services listed in the 2000–69999 code services. Modifier 63 should not be appended to any CPT codes listed in the evaluation and management services, anesthesia, radiology, pathology/laboratory, or medicine sections.
66	**Surgical team:** Under some circumstances, highly complex procedures (requiring the concomitant services of several physicians, often of different specialties, plus other highly skilled, specially trained personnel and various types of complex equipment) are carried out under the surgical team concept. Such circumstances may be identified by each participating physician with the addition of the modifier 66 to the basic procedure number used for reporting services.
73	**Discontinued outpatient hospital/ambulatory surgery center (ASC) procedure prior to the administration of anesthesia:** Due to extenuating circumstances or those that threaten the well-being of the patient, the physician may cancel a surgical or diagnostic procedure subsequent to the patient's surgical preparation (including sedation when provided, and being taken to the room where the procedure is to be performed), but prior to the administration of anesthesia (local, regional block(s) or general). Under these circumstances, the intended service that is prepared for but canceled can be reported by its usual procedure number and the addition of the modifier 73 or by use of the separate five-digit modifier code 09973. **Note:** The elective cancellation of a service prior to the administration of anesthesia and/or surgical preparation of the patient should not be reported. For physician reporting of a discontinued procedure, see modifier 53.
74	**Discontinued outpatient hospital/ambulatory surgery center (ASC) procedure after administration of anesthesia:** Due to extenuating circumstances or those due to extenuating circumstances or those that threaten the well-being of the patient, the physician may terminate a surgical or diagnostic procedure after the administration of anesthesia (local, regional block(s), general) or after the procedure was started (incision made,

Chapter 10: Modifier Descriptors

intubation started, scope inserted, etc.). Under these circumstances, the procedure started but terminated can be reported by its usual procedure number and the addition of the modifier 74. **Note:** The elective cancellation of a service prior to the administration of anesthesia and/or surgical preparation of the patient should not be reported. For physician reporting of a discontinued procedure, see modifier 53.

76   **Repeat procedure by same physician:** The physician may need to indicate that a procedure or service was repeated subsequent to the original procedure or service. This circumstance may be reported by adding the modifier 76 to the repeated procedure/service.

77   **Repeat procedure by another physician:** The physician may need to indicate that a basic procedure or service performed by another physician had to be repeated. This situation may be reported by adding modifier 77 to the repeated procedure/service.

78   **Return to the operating room for a related procedure during the postoperative period:** The physician may need to indicate that another procedure was performed during the postoperative period of the initial procedure. When this subsequent procedure is related to the first, and requires the use of the operating room, it may be reported by adding the modifier 78 to the related procedure. (For repeat procedures on the same day, see 76.)

79   **Unrelated procedure or service by the same physician during the postoperative period:** The physician may need to indicate that the performance of a procedure or service during the postoperative period was unrelated to the original procedure. This circumstance may be reported by using the modifier 79. (For repeat procedures on the same day, see 76).

80   **Assistant surgeon:** Surgical assistant services may be identified by adding the modifier 80 to the usual procedure number(s).

81   **Minimum assistant surgeon:** Minimum surgical assistant services are identified by adding the modifier 81 to the usual procedure number(s).

82   **Assistant surgeon (when qualified resident surgeon not available):** The unavailability of a qualified resident surgeon is a prerequisite for use of modifier 82 appended to the usual procedure code number(s) or by use of the separate five-digit modifier code 09982.

90   **Reference (outside) laboratory:** When laboratory procedures are performed by a party other than the treating or reporting physician, the procedure may be identified by adding the modifier 90 to the usual procedure number or by use of the separate five-digit modifier code 09990.

91   **Repeat clinical diagnostic laboratory test:** In the course of treatment of the patient, it may be necessary to repeat the same laboratory test on the same day to obtain subsequent (multiple) test results. Under these circumstances, the laboratory test performed can be identified by its usual procedure number and the addition of the modifier 91. **Note:** This modifier may not be used when tests are rerun to confirm initial results; due to testing

©2003 Ingenix, Inc.
CPT only ©2003 American Medical Association. All Rights Reserved.

problems with specimens or equipment; or for any other reason when a normal, one-time, reportable result is all that is required. This modifier may not be used when other code(s) describe a series of test results (e.g., glucose tolerance tests, evocative/suppression testing). This modifier may only be used for laboratory test(s) performed more than once on the same day on the same patient.

99   **Multiple modifiers:** Under certain circumstances two or more modifiers may be necessary to completely delineate a service. In such situations modifier 99 should be added to the basic procedure, and other applicable modifiers may be listed as part of the description of the service.

Notes

Notes

Notes

Notes

Notes

Notes

Notes

Notes